*Modern*
Athletic Training

# *Modern*

# Athletic Training

**KEN RAWLINSON**
*Head Athletic Trainer*
*University of Oklahoma*

PRENTICE-HALL, INC., Englewood Cliffs, N. J.

Second printing... August, 1962
Third printing.... November, 1964

# The Book . . . and the Author

Athletic training as a profession has been undergoing a tremendous transition in the last decade. There has been a greater interest emphasized by the medical societies in the whole area of athletic trauma than at any other period in history.

The administrators and coaches of the nation's high schools, colleges, and universities are seeking better trained, more qualified personnel to fill new positions and to replace retiring staff members. There is a vast growing need to seek knowledge from the experienced trainer as a supplement to formal academic education. For many years, there was far too little written on the subject of athletic training. With the advance in complexity of the various sports, the coach is often asked to assume responsibility far beyond his limited training.

Every experienced trainer is frequently asked about his specific treatments of athletic injury by the young trainer or high school coach. In this book, Ken Rawlinson has clearly answered the questions as they applied to him concerning athletic conditioning, prevention of injury, recognition of severity, treatment of trauma, and rehabilitation of the athlete both mentally and physically.

Every once in a while a book is written with a sincere effort on the part of the author to give unselfishly of his knowledge. This is such a book.

For the high school coach who finds it necessary to handle his own training problems for the student trainer, the young trainer, or the veteran trainer, this book can be a ready reference.

Mr. Rawlinson has the knowledge, experience and authority to make this book a *must* for those individuals vitally interested in proper care of the athlete. His techniques have justly earned him the same national prominence as the Oklahoma teams he has served so efficiently.

WILLIAM E. NEWELL
*Head Athletic Trainer*
*Purdue University*

# N.A.T.A. Code of Ethics

## PREAMBLE—PURPOSE OF CODE—AUTHORIZATION

### (Adopted June 1957)

The outstanding characteristics of a profession is that its members are dedicated to rendering services to humanity. Financial gain or personal reward must be secondary. In choosing the athletic training profession the individual assumes obligations and responsibilities to conduct himself in accord with its ideals and standards. These are listed and emphasized in the CODE OF ETHICS. Any trainer who does not deem it necessary to comply with the principles set forth in this CODE should have no place in this profession.

Athletics have gained prominent ground in our educational institutions and are maintaining an important position in our American way of life. The members of the athletic training profession must be vigilant in carrying out their small, but very necessary and significant role in our national athletic program. It is for this reason that the Directors of the National Athletic Trainers Association, at the Annual Meeting (June 20, 1954) authorized the preparation of a CODE OF ETHICS.

In formulating and presenting this CODE, the Committee on Ethics recognizes and believes that unless the standards and principles which this instrument represents are accepted whole-heartedly, it will be ineffective in solving our problems.

The reputation of any profession depends to a great degree upon the manner and conduct of its members in living up to the spirit and letter that its code of ethics represents. Ethics is generally defined as a science of moral duty, or making the right actions relative to ideal principles. Let it always be said that all members of this trainers' association will understand and apply the principles enumerated in this CODE, and make every effort to do the right thing at the right time to the best of their ability and judgment.

The primary purpose of this CODE is to clarify the ethical and approved professional practices as distinguished from those which might prove harmful and detrimental. Its secondary purpose is to instill into its members the value and importance of the athletic trainer's role in the entire athletic field.

## ENFORCEMENT

It is suggested that the Committee on Ethics be empowered to investigate all violations of the CODE which are brought to their attention. It is the duty of this Committee to collect all data pertaining to any reported violation, consider all sides of any controversial issue, and then forward a report of their findings and recommendations to the Board of Directors for final action.

It is further suggested that a written report of any unethical conduct be sent directly to the Chairman of The Board of Directors.

## OBJECTIVES

Among the stated objectives of the National Athletic Trainers Association are the following:

"The advancement, encouragement, and improvement of the athletic training profession in all its phases . . . develop further the ability of each of its members . . . provide a means for a free exchange of ideas within the profession . . . promote good fellowship among the members."
(Art. II By-Laws)

---

## ARTICLE I—BASIC PRINCIPLES

When a man becomes a member of the athletic training profession, he assumes a certain obligation and responsibilities to the following:

(1) Athletics in its broadest sense
(2) Players
(3) Physicians and Medical Advisors
(4) Parents
(5) Administrative Officials
(6) Coaches
(7) Fellow Trainers

The essential basic principles in this CODE OF ETHICS of the NATA are HONESTY, INTEGRITY, and LOYALTY. Athletic trainers who reflect these characteristics will be a credit to the Association, the institution they represent and to themselves. Such conduct will bring respect from all the people listed in the following sections.

### SEC. 1  ATHLETICS IN GENERAL

An athletic trainer should do all in his power and ability for all branches of athletics and show no discrimination in his interests or efforts.

### SEC. 2  PLAYERS

Each and every member of an athletic squad is a potential varsity player and should be treated without favoritism or partiality. An athletic trainer can wield a great amount of good influence on his charges by the proper conduct and use of good judgment in dealing with the various personalities and characters.

In prevention and treatment of injuries, the trainer must be very thorough in carrying out the accepted procedures and instructions. Any carelessness or laxity on the part of the trainer in his responsibility to the players in his charge is a breach of ethical practice.

### SEC. 3  PHYSICIANS AND MEDICAL ADVISORS

The athletic trainer should cooperate completely with the team physician or any other Medical Advisor assigned to the organization. The trainer must carry out the minute details of the doctor's orders, but not overstep his bound. Under no circumstances shall a trainer do medical or surgical procedures without specific instruction and consent of the physician in charge. Any deviation from the orders of the doctor, or failure to cooperate shall be considered unethical conduct.

## SEC. 4  PARENTS

In most every instance, a player on any athletic team is the parents' pride and joy. It is the responsibility of the trainer, by his conduct and interest, to assure all parents of the boys in his care that they are being properly cared for in every manner that is possible.

## SEC. 5  ADMINISTRATIVE OFFICIALS

It is the athletic trainer's responsibility to create a harmonious relationship between himself and all administrative officials. Suggestions and ideas should be freely discussed, but any controversial matters should be taken care of confidentially on a friendly basis. Decisions, business procedures and established standards should be given complete support by the trainer.

## SEC. 6  COACHES

There should be a close harmonious relationship between the trainer and all coaches based on mutual respect. Co-operation must be the key note—between coaches and training department in maintaining esprit-de-corps, proper conditioning of athletes, prevention methods, treatment of injuries, decisions relative to welfare of player and in every way possible for the good of all concerned.

## SEC. 7  FELLOW TRAINERS

The relationship of the trainers is partially set forth in the objectives. However, it should be stated further that in the process of extending courtesies and assisting our fellow trainers, we should abstain from so-called "second guessing" them in the care and treatment of their charges. Any suggestions should be given, or taken, in the spirit of constructive cooperation. Any trainer who by his conduct or derogatory comments discredits or lowers the dignity of members of his profession is guilty of a breach of ethics. Any report of unethical conduct should go through the proper channels and be kept within the confines of this association.

## ARTICLE II—CONDUCT—ATTITUDES—ACTIONS

The elements and subject matter in the following sections are of an abstract nature but are definitely to be considered in the realm of the athletic responsibilities and obligations.

### SEC. 1   SCHOLARSHIP

A fundamental responsibility of the trainer in an educational institution is to promote and inspire scholastic achievement. This may be accomplished by suggestions, example, and arranging study periods and tutoring.

### SEC. 2   TESTIMONIALS AND ENDORSEMENTS

When an athletic trainer accepts an offer for an endorsement of commercial items and commodities, he must realize that the offer is being made mainly because he is a successful representative of the training profession. In all endorsements where the training profession and the trainer's name are included, the phrasing and text of the testimonial should be such that it does not bring discredit to athletics in general, or to the training profession. Accepting money, or anything of material value for an endorsement of any item which is not in keeping with the highest principles and traditions of the athletic training profession, shall be considered unethical.

### SEC. 3   PUBLIC RELATIONS AND PUBLICATIONS

The ideal situation is for the director of publicity to handle all releases to the press. However, if the trainer is authorized to answer questions of newswriters and commentators, and provides them with news about the players, good judgment should be the keynote. Answer direct questions honestly, or not at all. If there is a possibility that an honest answer might be misleading or involve a detrimental interpretation, good judgment may prompt a "no comment", answer. Sports writers, broadcasters, and commentators should be treated with courtesy, honesty, and respect.

Magazine articles, newspaper columns and any information for the public press, radio and television given by a member of the training profession is strictly that individual's responsibilty. Good judgment should indicate that no statements be said or written that reflect discredit to athletics in general or the athletic training profession. Any professional problems that arise should be settled within the Association, and not in the public press.

### SEC. 4   PRE-GAME—GAME—POST-GAME ACTIVITIES

Meet the visiting trainer and offer any available services that he may desire. Meet and exchange greetings with the manager and coach. Make arrangements for any medical assistance that is necessary for the visiting team during the entire time they are your guests. During the warm-up period and game, carry on the training activities, but be as inconspicuous as possible. After the game, determine if there is any emergency service that the visiting team needs and give assistance in any way possible. Always have a respectful attitude to officials, visiting players, and coaches.

### SEC. 5   SPORTSMANSHIP

The athletic trainer is in a position to aid the coaches in instilling fair play and good sportsmanship in the players. Any athletic trainer who permits, condones, or defends unsportsmanlike practices which are dangerous to a player shall be considered guilty of a serious breach of ethics.

### THE ETHICS COMMITTEE

HOWARD WAITE, Chairman, University of Pittsburgh
STEPHEN WITKOWSKI, Wesleyan University, Conn.
MARTY BROUSSARD, Louisiana State University
JACK WILLIAMSON, University of California
ROBERT G. BRASHEAR, M.D. Advisory

# Table of Contents

*My main purpose in writing this book is to gather together the information, know-how, and techniques from my own experience and from what I have learned from so many gracious trainers and doctors in the past. I am deeply cognizant of and grateful for all their help and only hope that this book may be of value to present and future trainers.*

*Modern*
Athletic Training

# CHAPTER 1

# The Trainer in
# Modern Athletics

The background of athletic training is long and illustrious. It had its start with the ancient Greek and Roman athletic contests, as evidenced in our archeological museums. Artists of the time found much of their inspiration in scenes on the gymnasium, palestra, track, and field. Vases, our most important record, reflect the various phases of the life of the athlete. Bronze and marble sculptures, gems, and coins also add to our knowledge. Recorded on these vases are many instances of the aryballos (oil flask), strigil (instrument for removing oil and dust from the body after exercise), and sponges. Other specific scenes shown on vases include an attendant drawing a thorn from an athlete's foot, and two scenes entitled "Wrestlers with their trainer in the palestra." Another, perhaps the first recorded instance of a trainer instructing the principles of fair play, is entitled "Trainer beating with his stick a youth who is gouging his opponent's eye."

From the time the ancient Greeks pitched their tents on the plains of the Elis in the dim centuries of the past and brought together the young men of their land in the first of all Olympic games, until their modern revival in 1896 and down through recent times, the trainer has been an important factor in keeping the athlete in condition for top performance.

Through the years the duties and qualifications of the trainers have changed in the same manner that the three R's of "reading, 'riting, and 'rithmetic" have changed to the present "rockets, radiation, and rock and roll." The crude methods of the old-time trainers have become a thing of the past. The day of "the rubber," the know-it-all jack-of-all-trades and master-of-none, is over. Following World War I, the athletic trainer as a specialist in the prevention of injury made his appearance in intercollegiate athletics. It was at this time, 1917, that Dr. S. E. Bilik published the first text devoted exclusively to athletic training and the treatment of athletic injuries (5, 6). Other excellent publications have appeared since (7-10). (Numbers in parentheses refer to entries in bibliography at end of chapter).

The trainer today must have a sound understanding of the human body and be a keen and unbiased observer of the body in action. He must know a good deal about physiology, kinesiology, psychology, hygiene, massage, conditioning, therapeutic exercise, diet, and the various modalities of physical therapy. In addition, he is the father confessor of the squad.

In a recent study "Red" Burnett, Trainer at Utah State University (11), found that very little research had been done on the history and background of athletic training. He further stated that there were many books and pamphlets on training methods but none that elaborated the duties of the trainer or what his qualifications should be. Fortunately, steps have been taken by the National Athletic Trainers Association (N.A.T.A.) to remedy this situation.

This organization was founded in Kansas City, Missouri, on June 24, 1950. Its objectives are:

1. The advancement, encouragement, and improvement of the athletic training profession in all its phases and promotion of a better working relationship among those persons interested in the problems of training.

2. To develop further the ability of each of its members.

3. To better serve the common interest of its members by providing means for a free exchange of ideas within the profession.

4. To enable members to become better acquainted personally through casual good fellowship.

At the present time there are six classes of membership: active, associate, allied, advisory, honorary, and retired. As of June,

1960, there was a total membership of 733. Authority and responsibility for the Association is vested in nine directors who represent geographical districts of the United States or athletic conferences previously organized. One of the district directors is annually selected as chairman of the board.

Since 1950 the N.A.T.A. has held an Annual Meeting in June of each year. They have all been well-attended and have featured as speakers outstanding medical, surgical, and orthopedic specialists of the United States. Warm approval of the aims and purposes of the Association has been forthcoming from many leaders in various fields of medicine.

In June, 1955, at Boston, the Board of Directors of the N.A.T.A. appointed a Committee on Professional Advancement consisting of thirteen athletic trainers and five medical advisors (Drs. R. G. Brashear, J. S. Feurig, D. H. O'Donoghue, W. D. Paul, and E. T. Smith). The committee was instructed to develop an educational curriculum that would be acceptable to the colleges and universities of the nation. This committee, after three years of study, presented a proposed curriculum to the membership at large for comment in 1958. This included: (1) a curriculum that would give the individual the broadest teaching certificate possible; (2) a curriculum of pre-physical therapy courses that would be accepted by any American Medical Association-approved physical therapy school; (3) a curriculum to prepare men in the management and prevention of athletic injuries. At the present time, only one institution in the United States, the University of Indiana, is offering a bachelor of science degree in athletic training. No doubt in years to come, if the aforementioned curriculum is accepted, the standards of future trainers will be raised. The committee is also exploring the possibility of formal alliance of the N.A.T.A. with the medical profession.

In September, 1956, the N.A.T.A. started publishing its own quarterly journal, covering new methods, recent developments, and other matters pertinent to training and of interest to trainers.

In 1957, the N.A.T.A. became an affiliated member of the National Collegiate Athletic Association and a Group "E" member of the United States Olympic Committee.

In addition to the N.A.T.A., each of the nine regional trainers' associations are self-governing through their own specific constitutions and by-laws. In their relation with the national organization, regional associations are under the jurisdiction of the N.A.T.A. constitution and by-laws.

In 1957 the Council of the National Collegiate Athletic Association authorized the appointment of a Committee on Sports Injuries and Safety. The purposes of this committee are:

1. To collect and develop pertinent information regarding the prevention and treatment of sports injuries and utilization of sound safety measures at the college level.

2. To disseminate such information as might be appropriately brought to the attention of the member institutions of the N.C.A.A.

3. To recommend the establishment of policies and standards by N.C.A.A. rules and tournament committees, or the Association as a whole, designed to better the safety factor in college athletics.

This committee is selected by the N.C.A.A. It consists of the following: Director of Athletics, Head Football Coach, Dean of a School of Physical Education, Physiologist, an American Medical Association representative, and a Trainer.

To date, this committee has completed the following surveys: (1) A study of injuries to the head, face, shoulder, neck, pelvis, knee, and ankle that were serious enough to necessitate a boy's missing a practice session or make it necessary to alter his daily practice routine. (2) A listing of standards for equipping and maintaining a training room for the prevention, treatment, and rehabilitation of athletic injuries. Both surveys were conducted by various trainers in the United States. Thus, athletic trainers in the United States, through organization, establishment of standards and participation in a program of inquiry, are achieving the status of a true paramedical profession.

The daily activities of the trainer are principally concerned with prevention of injury, treatment under medical direction and rehabilitation.

Most trainers spend more time on prevention of injuries than is commonly believed by the average layman or even by most school officials. It should be emphasized that treatment is only part of the trainer's duties and probably a less important part. The more injuries that can be prevented, the fewer there will be to treat and rehabilitate. Since an injured athlete is of no value to his team, his coach, or to himself from an athletic standpoint, the greatest concern must be with prevention of the injury which causes his disability.

A most important phase of prevention is the physical and mental conditioning of the squad. It must be a vital part of the program. Bob Shelton of the University of Illinois, in an address before the Illinois Association for Health, Physical Education and Recreation, made the following statement: "Conditioning is more important than skill, because conditioning helps prevent injuries and the best halfback in the world is of no value sitting on the bench." (See Chapter III)

Many factors go into the field of prevention. As a part of prevention, no person should be permitted to practice or participate in any sport until he has successfully passed a thorough physical examination. At the University of Oklahoma, we give our physical examinations on the so-called assembly line technique. Our team physician, doctors from the health service, and nurses give physical examinations at the student infirmary at 8:00 A.M. on the day before fall practice starts. Each doctor takes a station. The boys are given their record cards and they merely go from station to station. With the use of this technique, we have been able to give our varsity football squad its physical examinations in a relatively short period of time.

Along this same line, it is strongly recommended that a physician be on the bench at every contest. It may be necessary, in some localities, for various doctors to take turns; but, regardless of how it is done, a doctor can be rendering a service to his community by donating his services for a couple of evenings each year.

Prevention also includes surveys of dressing rooms, shower rooms, playing fields, and equipment, to eliminate all possible hazards. Many schools spend most of their money and all of their time maintaining a so-called perfect game-field—a field the spectators will see and the team will use four or five times a year. I would recommend that, more important, the *practice field,* which is used as much in a week as the game field is in a season, be kept in A-1 condition at all times.

Good equipment is an important factor in the prevention of injuries. Some schools make the same mistake with equipment as they do with their practice field. They spend the greater portion of their budget for some gaudy, fancy game-suit that is going to be worn only eight to ten times a year. It is my belief that a school should spend most of its money for the equipment that is worn daily—practice equipment. Although the budget is limited, one should warn against the purchasing of large quantities of second-rate equipment—otherwise, no player is properly protected. It is recommended instead that schools purchase the best even though the supply may be limited. Too much emphasis cannot be placed on a proper headgear. The modern, lightweight headgear is effective, but does little good if the suspension apparatus is not properly placed to keep the head from contact with the inside of the headgear (see Chapter XIII). Once good equipment is supplied, the trainer and coach should insist that, in order to compete, the player wear the equipment that has been prepared for him.

At least a weekly check of each player's equipment should be made by the trainer or some other responsible person. Is the suspension in the headgear too loose? Are shoulder pads or hip pads broken? Are the pants too large so that the thigh pads are sliding? How are the shoe cleats? A single loose suspension string in the headgear can mean a severe concussion. The slipping of a thigh pad may result in a contusion (Charley horse) which can keep a player inactive for the rest of the season.

From time to time during the season, it is necessary to improvise or purchase special equipment to protect a special injury. A fracture-glove may be necessary to protect a hand injury, a pair of "Big Boy" shoulder pads to protect a bruised shoulder, or a pair of "Peel Blocker" hip pads to protect an iliac crest. It may be necessary to build up a pair of regular shoulder pads with sponge rubber or plastic to protect a bruise or separation, or to use a folded towel around the neck to prevent recurring neck sprains or nerve contusions.

It is also necessary in fielding a team to do a considerable amount of preventive and protective taping. This will be discussed in the following chapters.

If the injury cannot be prevented, the first important step is early detection of its nature and degree. The best time to examine an athlete is at the time of the injury. Too often the injury is packed in ice, or strapped until the next day. This is a dangerous practice. The trainer should work hand-in-hand with the team physician. They should function as a team with the same set of rules and signals and the same objective—the complete rehabilitation of the player. It must be kept in mind that there are several conditions which make the treatment of the athlete quite different from that of the ordinary patient. Dr. E. T. Smith of Houston, Texas, lists them as: (1) He is, or should be, strong, and in excellent physical condition. (2) He is young, and his healing and recuperative power is above average. (3) He has an incentive to get well, will cooperate to the fullest extent, and will tolerate early rehabilitative procedures. Because of these factors it is usually possible to get an athlete back into competition in a much shorter period of time than it is for an average workingman to return to his job.

Rehabilitative exercises should be started as soon as possible after an injury. In fact, it is advisable to continue exercising other portions of the body even though the injured part must of necessity be immobilized. It is much better to prevent atrophy than to relieve it. Obviously some exercises will be more suitable than others for a specific situation, and they must all be proportioned to the degree of disability of the individual player and gradually increased as he improves. It should be emphasized again that the player as a whole should be treated, and not simply the injured part. It is only the unusual injury that will not permit active exercise of other parts of the body from the first day. Recovery must be complete. One hundred per cent rehabilitation must be the goal.

A related problem with which the trainer, coach, or team physician is confronted is the player who is afraid of injury. It is necessary to convince him that if he gets himself in the proper condition he will not be subject to injury.

The trainer is in a unique position to build confidence by convincing the player that if he is in top physical condition, uses his equipment properly, is adequately warmed up, follows the coach's instructions precisely, and plays with "carefree abandon" and no hesitation, it is very unlikely that he will be hurt.

If confidence cannot be instilled and he remains "gun shy," he should be advised to drop out of the sport in the interest of his own safety.

It is encouraging to note that there are fewer serious injuries every year. This improvement can be explained in part by the fact that there are more qualified men in the field of conditioning, that better equipment has been designed and is being used, and that everyone is becoming increasingly concerned about the prevention of injuries. It has been said that, in the past, coaches were concerned about getting a team on the field, but now they are vitally interested in keeping a team on the field. An adequate training program is one of the best means to accomplish this end.

It is a recognized fact that many schools cannot hire a full-time trainer. I would suggest that these schools take into consideration one of the following—hire a teacher-trainer, a qualified college graduate who has worked as an assistant trainer in college and who can also teach in the school system; (this plan is in effect quite extensively throughout Texas). It may even be possible in larger cities for two or three schools to hire a full-time trainer and establish a centralized training room in which all athletes could be taken care of.

If neither of the above methods are feasible, I would suggest that each school appoint a sincerely interested boy as a student trainer. Put him in charge of the training room, training equipment and first aid measures both on and off the field, but under the direct supervision of the coach. It would be advisable that the student trainer have no duties other than those connected with his training work. This student assistant will be able to perform numerous services which will give the coach more time in his already over-crowded schedule. To better educate our student trainers in the principles of first aid, the Cramer Chemical Co., Gardner, Kansas, has inaugurated a free summer correspondence course for all student trainers who are interested in enrolling, (one from each school).

Following are a few suggestions for student trainers, (courtesy of the Cramer Chemical Co.):

1. Be the first man on the job and the last one to leave.

2. Keep your training room clean and neat but don't spend time housekeeping when there are players needing attention.

3. Let the *coach* make and enforce rules. They are his responsibility, not yours.

4. Put your supplies away before going home at night. Get them out in the morning, after you have put the room in order.

5. Find things to do in slack moments.

6. Prepare a "want list" of needed supplies. Make this a daily practice. It will be the coach's responsibility to order them if he feels they are necessary.

7. Always keep your First Aid Kit properly packed for field and trip use.

8. Your hands are your most important tools. Keep them clean. Keep your nails trimmed and clean under them before and after each day's work.

9. A special uniform isn't necesary, but dress neatly. Prove you are worthy of the respect of the squad, and you will get it.

10. When you are in doubt, ask the coach.

11. Always be loyal to the coach. When things get tough, as they often do, prove that you are a part of the team.

12. Plan trips with the coach. Let him advise you on extra supplies that may be needed.

13. Don't get involved in local quarterback club discussions. Let the coach handle the news on player condition and prospects.

14. Your job is to lessen the physical and mental load of the coach, and he will be surprised at how well you can do it if you work at it properly.

15. Don't experiment with new methods until you have learned the merits and disadvantages of the old ones.

16. The only time you or anyone else can decide whether or not an injury is "minor," is after it has healed.

17. You may not have as good a training room as your neighbor but do the best you can with what you have. Don't acquire the habit of being a complainer or grumbler.

18. Don't have pets or favorites. Every star and scrub should rank equally in the training room, unless the coach instructs you differently. (Today's scrub may be next year's star).

19. Close to 60% of your time will be spent preventing injury. Thoroughness will save time.

20. During practice or a game, pay particular attention to those you know have some sort of injury and check every player at half-time or as occasion permits.

21. Don't be guilty of letting a "little knowledge become dangerous." The coach and team or school physician must be responsible for the athlete's welfare.

22. Use your ears and eyes to improve the efficiency of your hands. In other words, read and observe what other trainers and coaches are doing.

I would strongly recommend that a physician be available at all contests. If each school were to provide a physician at all of its home contests, it would not be necessary for the physicians to travel with the visiting team.

REFERENCES

1. Thorwaldsen Museum, Copenhagen, No. 112; and Museum für antike Kleinhunst, Munich, No. 2344.
2. Altes Museum, Berlin, No. 2180.
3. Altes Museum, Berlin, No. 2159.
4. Metropolitan Museum of Art, *Greek Athletics* (3rd. ed.), New York, 1933. Plandome Press.
5. Bilik, S. E., *The Trainers' Bible* (8th revised ed.), New York, 1947. T. J. Reed Co.
6. Bilik, S. E., *Athletic Training and the Treatment of Athletic Injuries* (3rd. ed.), New York, 1923. Atsco Press.
7. Cramer, F., Boughton, L. L. and Cramer, C., *A Training Room Manual*, Gardner, Kan., 1944. Cramer Co.
8. Dolan, J. P., *Treatment and Prevention of Athletic Injuries* (1st ed.), Danville, Ill., 1955. Interstate Co.
9. Thorndike, A., *Athletic Injuries, Prevention, Diagnosis and Treatment* (3rd. ed.), Philadelphia, 1948. Lea & Febiger.
10. Morehouse, L. F. and Rasch, P. J., *Scientific Basis of Athletic*

*Training* (1st. ed.), Philadelphia, 1958. W. B. Saunders Co.

11. Burnett, R., Personal communication.
12. Secretary's report. Second Annual Convention and Clinic of the National Athletic Trainers' Association. Kansas City, Mo., June, 1951.
13. O'Donoghue, D. H. and Rawlinson, K., "The Prevention and Treatment of Athletic Injuries." J. Oklahoma M. A., 49: 219-221, 255-258, 263-264, 3-2-306, 310, 1956.
14. Quigley, T. B., Cox, J. and Murphy, J., "Protective Wrapping for the Ankle." J.A.M.A., 132: 924, 1946.
15. Hanley, D. F., Personal communication.
16. Rawlinson, K. B., "Symposium on Sports Injuries." American Journal of Surgery, 98:337, 1959.

# CHAPTER II

# The Training Room

It is a known fact that every school cannot have an ideal training room, but every school can have a clean training room.

## CLEANLINESS MUST BE THE KEYNOTE

It is extremely hard to specify the actual equipment and supplies as there is such a difference in the size of schools, their budgets, and their needs. Any equipment and supplies purchased should be approved by the team physician. Work hand-in-hand with him and use nothing of which he does not approve. Make the best of what you have and perhaps sometime in the future the room can be enlarged and more equipment added. Just remember that the most important thing in the training room is the person who is in charge of the operation—the trainer himself.

Following are some considerations which should be taken into account in setting up the training room:

A. Location
  1. Adjacent to athletes' dressing room.
  2. Bathroom adjoining.
  3. As close as possible to exercise and games area.

B. General Plan
  1. Painted a light, pleasant color (waterproof and washable).
  2. Good ventilation, outlet fans.
  3. Adequate heat (air conditionnig not advisable).
  4. Adequate fluorescent overhead lighting.
  5. Sufficient electrical outlets at least 4 feet above floor.

6. Linoleum or tile floor.
7. Telephone.
8. Outside windows (bottoms 5 feet from floor).
9. If only one room is available, it should be large enough to contain at least:
   a. Training tables—1—20 athletes (74″ x 24″ x 30″ to 34″).
   b. Taping tables—1—20 athletes (36″ x 24″ x 30″ to 34″).
   c. Sink with hot and cold water.
   d. Essential physical therapy equipment (under equipment).
   e. Area for rehabilitation equipment (under equipment).
   f. Desk for trainer and physician.
   g. File for records.
   h. Shelves and cupboards for storage.
   i. Refrigerator.
   j. Table for sterilizer and supplies.
   k. Foot powder bench (preferably in dressing room).
   l. Chairs or benches.
   m. Trash containers.
10. If more than one room is available, consideration should be given to these needs:
   a. Physical therapy and rehabilitation room.
   b. Office for trainer and physician, with examining table.
   c. Steam room.
   d. Water-cooling unit for sprains, etc.
   e. X-ray room.
   f. Bulletin board.

C. Equipment
  1. Physical Therapy
   a. Whirlpool baths (one large and one small).
   b. Infra-red lamps.
   c. Diathermy.
   d. Hydrocollator.
   e. Ultrasonic.
   f. Medcollator.
   g. Electric heat pads.
   h. Combination massage and heat pad.
   i. Ultra-violet lamp.
   j. Paraffin bath.
   k. Electric massage table.
   l. Hand vibrators.

2. Rehabilitation Equipment
    a. Progressive resistance-exercise equipment (weights, pulleys, leg weight table, Logan knee strengthener, stationary bicycle, shoulder wheel, etc.).
    b. Traction unit.
    c. Hanging bar (shoulders, etc.).
    d. Mats.
3. Medical and Trainers
    a. Stretchers.
    b. Crutches (adjustable) and canes.
    c. Splints (finger, arm, leg, etc.). Wood, ring type, metal and alumafoam.
    d. Oxygen unit.
    e. Spotlight and magnifying glass.
    f. Ice bags.
    g. Electric and blade razors.
    h. Bandage scissors.
    i. Gilcrest tape-cutter.
    j. Ankle-wrap roller.
    k. Hair dryer.
    l. Bag for field use.
    m. Tourniquet.
    n. Flashlight.
    o. Thermometer.
    p. Music.
    q. Basins.
    r. As requested by the team physician.
        1. Surgical instruments and sutures.
        2. Syringes and needles.
    s. Sterilizers.
    t. Wheel-chair.
    u. Portable training table.

D. Supplies (partial listing)
    1. Sterile Dressings
        a. Gauze pads (2 by 2 in., 3 by 3 in.).
        b. Band Aids—plastic and elastic.
        c. Telfa pads (various sizes).
        d. Gel-foam (small strips).
        e. Kling bandage (2 by 3 in. width).
        f. Non-adherent oil-impregnated mesh (4 by 4 in.).
    2. Non-sterile dressings
        a. Gauze roller bandage (1 in., 2 in., 3 in.).
        b. Absorbent cotton (lb. rolls).

      c. Combine roll.
      d. Gauze pads (2 by 2 in. and 3 by 3 in.).
      e. Ankle wraps (72-yard rolls and cut to desired length).
      f. Elastic bandages (2 in., 3 in., and 4 in.).
      g. Triangular bandage.
      h. Tubegauze.
3. Adhesive Tape
      a. Regular (½ in., 1 in., 1½ in. and 2 in.).
      b. Elastic (2 in. and 3 in.).
      c. Moleskin adhesive.
4. Capsules
      a. Ammonia capsules.
      b. Gar-capsules.
5. Ointments

      a. Cramergesic.
      b. Atomic Balm.
      c. Red Hot.
      d. Cold Cream.
      e. Ergophene.
      f. Firm Grip.
      g. Foot Ointment.
      h. Strawberry Ointment.
      i. Inhalant.
      j. Pragmatar.
      k. Mexsana Skin Cream.
      l. Pazo.
      m. Sun Glare Black.
      n. Spectrocin Ophthalmic Ointment.
      o. Sopronol.
      p. Unguentine.
      q. Vaseline.
      r. Zinc Oxide.

6. Padding
      a. Felt (⅜ in., ¼ in.).
      b. Plastic.
      c. Foam rubber.
      d. Corn plasters.
      e. Bruise pads.
      f. Foot pads.
7. Powders
      a. Foot and Body powder.
      b. Boric Acid.
      c. Epsom Salts.
      d. Rosin.
8. Solutions

      a. Alcohol 70%.
      b. Iso Quin.
      c. Athletic Liniment.
      d. Atomic Rub Down.
      e. Am-Spray Ammonia.
      f. Fungo-Spray.
      g. Ace Adherent.
      h. Calamine.
      i. Oil of cloves.
      j. Collodion.
      k. Cough syrup.

l. Cuprex.
m. Eye wash.
n. Tape Remover.
o. Ivy Dry.
p. Iotanagen.
q. Mineral Oil.
r. Nitrogen Spray and Liquid.
s. Merthiolate.
t. Athletic Soap.
u. Kaopectate.
v. Pepto-Bismol.
w. Milk of Magnesia.
x. Mycozol.
y. Gym-Fresh-Ner Spray.
z. Neo-Synephrine ½%.
aa. Peroxide, Hydrogen.
bb. Q.D.A. Spray and Liquid.
cc. Stringent Gargle.
dd. Sun Screen.
ee. Sprahalant.
ff. Tuf-Skin Spray and Liquid.
gg. Wintergreen.
hh. Firm Grip Spray.
ii. Kleen-Ball.
jj. Spirits of Peppermint.

9. Tablets

a. Aspirin 5 gr.
b. A.B.A. Cold Tabs.
c. Cascara.
d. Dextrose-B$^1$.
e. Rhinitis.
f. Salt-Impregnated 10 gr.
g. Titralac.
h. Hi-Score "C."
i. Butterfly (alkaline).
j. Empirin.

10. Miscellaneous

a. Cotton Tip applicators.
b. Elastic thigh caps.
c. Elastic knee caps.
d. Cast material.
e. Braces.
f. Tongue depressors.
g. Rib belt—6 in.
h. Face bars.
i. Tooth protectors.
j. Atomizers.
k. Towels.
l. Blankets.
m. Sheets.
n. Fire extinguisher.
o. Heel cups.
p. Toothache wax.
q. Resusitube (J & J).

11. Others as suggested by the team physician

The whirlpool bath is one of the safest and most effective physical-therapeutic agents in use today. It can be used in treating practically any type of injury: sprains, strains, contusions, bone injuries, post fractures, bursitis, circulatory disturbances, synovities, painful joints, scar tissue, nerve injuries, adhesions, arthritis, etc.

Several factors influence the length of time for each treatment. In treating an extremity, the average length of time is twenty minutes; if the patient is submerged to the hips, the average treatment time is 12 to 15 minutes; if the entire body is submerged, the treatment time should be from five to ten minutes.

Insofar as water temperature is concerned, remember that the more acute the injury, the lower the intensity of heat—heat will cause swelling to an injured area. We abide by the following rules in regard to the water temperature in our whirlpools:

New injury or injury with swelling—under 100 degrees.
Injury at least 3-4 days old (little swelling)—100 to 106 degrees.
Old, chronic injury—106 to 110 degrees.

If considerable swelling is present at times, we place an elastic wrap over the area before putting it into the whirlpool.

As a safety precaution, the whirlpool should be grounded and have a working thermometer. Sapping of an individual's strength is related to the length of treatment and the temperature of the water. Observe the boy closely after a treatment because of a tendency of some to become lightheaded.

I consider the whirlpool and the infra-red lamp the first pieces of therapy equipment which should be placed in a training room.

It is recognized that many schools cannot afford some of the above therapeutic equipment. However, it is possible to improvise and make therapy equipment which will aid in the treatment of athletic injuries. Some of the home-made equipment or relatively inexpensive equipment which have proven of value are:

1. Contrast baths—very effective in stimulating circulation to the extremities. Fill one bucket with hot water (104-110 degrees) and one with cold water (45-50 degrees). Alternately submerge the extremity into the buckets, starting with hot and ending with hot if there is no swelling. Where there is swelling, end with cold. The ratio will vary. Ratios (in minutes) are

hot to cold 10-1, 6-4, 5-3, 3-1 (best for most injuries). Another phase of the contrast bath is to wrap the extremity with an elastic wrap over a sponge and place in the whirlpool for two minutes (hot) and then ten seconds in a cold tub. Still another phase is to use the garden hose on the injured area and alternate the hot and cold water according to the above recommendations.

2.  Homemade whirlpools.

3.  Shower—adjust the nozzle so that there is a forceful, direct spray, especially good on neck, shoulders and back.

4.  Hot towels.

5.  Hot-tub soaking.

6.  Hot-water bottle.

7.  Ice.

8.  Water-cooling box.

9.  Salt glow—make a salt paste and massage the body and follow with a hot shower. Good for fatigue and staleness.

10.  Percussion douche (garden hose)—start 10-15 feet away with warm water (105 degrees) and plenty of pressure. Play the water stream along the back, sides and front of the body, break the stream with fingers over tender areas. Repeat with cold water.

11.  Chemical heat pads.

12.  Hydrocollator. Purchase the hydrocollator pads and make your own heating unit.

13.  Homemade lamps.

14.  Paraffin bath. Three parts of paraffin (jelly wax) to one part of vaseline in a homemade container.

15  Steam bath.

# CHAPTER III

# Conditioning Athletes' Bodies

For top performance, body conditioning is absolutely necessary. A conditioned boy is less susceptible to injuries. Conditioning affects:

1. Ability to play.
2. Mental attitude.
3. Determination.
4. Teamwork.
5. Spirit.

Many fail to make the team because they do not have the desire. They will not pay the price to get themselves into shape both physically and mentally. Mental conditioning is a phase often overlooked, but it is very vital. Many athletes do not think it is important, but it goes hand-in-hand with physical conditioning. If an athlete is going to be great, he must have both. The long-time and honored track coach at the University of Oklahoma, John Jacobs, made the following statement in 1958 which I believe summarizes the situation. He stated that "Coaching and mental condition are important. Mental attitude is far more vital than anyone realizes. Breaking the four minute barrier was largely mental. It's like the first time you go off the highboard in a swimming pool."

## CONDITIONING AT OKLAHOMA

The conditioning program for the fall season at the University of Oklahoma begins at the close of spring football practice (approximately the middle of April). This portion of the conditioning program must be carried on by the athlete himself. He cannot be expected to do this without proper direction and instruction. It is our firm conviction that if athletes have the desire to be great, they must be, and are, willing to pay the price to help accomplish their goal.

Red Sanders, the late head football coach at U.C.L.A., once made the statement that football is forty per cent ability and sixty per cent physical condition and mental attitude. Tom Harmon, former Michigan All-American and presently a sportscaster, went Red one better on a recent radio show when he stated that football these days is ninety per cent mental and physical preparation. It all boils down to the axiom that no team is better than its physical condition. Your objective must be to get your team, as a whole and as individuals, physically stronger and tougher than your opponent. You must impress on your players that many fail to make the team for no other reason than that they are unwilling to pay the price to get themselves in tip-top physical condition.

### BASIC PRINCIPLES OF RUNNING

An important phase of conditioning is running. Every athlete should learn how to run correctly. Anyone can be taught to run a little faster, if he has the desire. Following are a few suggestions:

1. Relax. The body must be supple to attain best performance.

2. Run on balls of the feet.

3. Point the toes straight ahead. You lose at least one-half inch on each step if toes are not straight ahead.

4. Run in a straight line. It is the shortest distance between two points.

5. Develop your proper stride. The average stride is the height of your body. Lengthen your stride as much as possible but do not overstride. It is worse than an understride.

6. Running angle is important; body leaning, head up, ankles, hips, shoulders and head in a straight line. Do not bend too far backward. You should be in the proper running angle and with the proper stride 12-15 yards from the starting point.

7.  Arm action is very important; opposite arm and leg move in unison. Keep arm relaxed and shoot uppercuts to height of shoulder and not beyond center of body. Bring arm back so hand does not go beyond crest of hip, a relaxed piston-like movement.

Short sprints develop speed.

Distance-running develops endurance.

Running in circles and figure eights strengthens ankles, knees, hips, and backs.

The yearly conditioning program at the University of Oklahoma is as follows: (Take into consideration that we work on rehabilitation the year around.)

APRIL—MAY:

Workout three times a week. Run, tennis, golf, handball, track, weights, and exercises. Assign weights for September weigh-in.

JUNE:

Run two or three times a week, distance-running plus daily exercises. (See Below)

JULY:

Run three to four days a week, distance-running plus a few sprints and daily exercises. (See Below)

AUGUST:

Increase the tempo in everything. Workout five to seven days a week, with emphasis on sprinting (properly warmed up), conditioning drills, and football drills.

DAILY EXERCISE GUIDE:

Do five exercises per day for six days a week during the months of June and July. Increase the tempo in August. These exercises are set up specifically to reach every area of the body, and can be done daily in the athlete's room or back yard. He should start exercises by jumping rope.

MONDAY:

*Side Bender*—Position: Stand with feet apart, hands clasped overhead, arms straight. Bend sideward to the right, bending right knee and slowly going as far as possible. Repeat to left. Repeat ten times each side.

*Knee Stretcher*—Position: Stand with feet apart, knees slightly flexed and hands on outside of knees. Press knees together with hands. Knees offering resistance. Repeat outward twenty times.

*Shoulder Hang*—Position: Grasp an overhead crossbar, ladder, tree limb, etc., and hang elbows straight. Hang one minute, relax and repeat ten times. Especially good for boys with A-C, muscular, or nerve shoulder trouble. (If shoulder will permit, walk hand-over-hand across overhead ladder).

*Hurdle Spread*—Position: Sit in hurdle position with right leg forward. Bend trunk forward and touch right foot with both hands. Repeat forty times, then extend left leg and repeat forty times.

TUESDAY:

*Groin Stretch*—Position: Stand with feet apart, hands on groin. Bend body obliquely to right and left (forward and backward). Stretch it out.

*Bicycle Ride*—Position: Support body on shoulders with elbows on ground and hands on hips supporting the body. Move feet and legs in motion necessary for riding a bicycle as rapidly as possible for count of forty. Repeat four to five times.

*Stomach Drill*—Position: Flat on back with hands under hips, with legs straight together, and toes pointed. Raise feet slowly with a slow count of ten until the legs are perpendicular to the ground, lower them slowly halfway and stop; here spread the legs and bring them together eight times, then lower legs to within six inches from the ground and repeat the spread eight times. Raise legs slowly to the perpendicular position and lower them to the ground very slowly. Repeat eight times.

*Leg Flexing*—Position: Sitting position. With both hands grasp left leg and pull knee up to ear. Relax and repeat with right leg. Repeat rapidly for count of 100.

WEDNESDAY:

*Wood Chopper*—Position: Stand with feet apart, trunk turned right, hands together and over right shoulder. In a chopping movement bring arms down vigorously between the legs. Uncoil over left shoulder and repeat. Repeat twenty times each side.

*Push Up or Push Up and Clap*—Position: Flat on stomach with toes dug in and hands flat on ground, clap hands and catch on hands without allowing body to contact ground. Repeat ten to fifteen times.

*Quarter Eagles*—Position: Feet width of shoulders, parallel, and heels on ground. Bend at knees so thighs are parallel to ground. Maintaining the above base jump ¼ turns to right and left.

*Belly Rock*—Position: Face down, hands back of neck. Raise head, chest and feet and rock back and forth seventy-five times.

Thursday:

*Trunk Twister*—Position: Stand with feet apart, hands clasped behind head and elbows back. Bend and bounce downward and simultaneously rotate trunk far to left. Recover and repeat to right. Repeat fifteen times to each side.

*All Fours*—Position: Face down. Weight on hands and feet, and walk forward, backward, sideward, etc. (crab walk—same exercise with back down).

*Burpee*—Position: Standing (1) Squat-position with hands on ground, elbows inside knees. Thrust feet and legs backward, weight supported on hands and toes. Return to squat-position, then to starting position. Repeat twenty times.

*Sit Up and Paw Dirt*—Position: Flat on back with arms extended overhead. Sit up, thrust arms forward and touch toes, knees straight. Return to starting position. Swing legs overhead until feet touch ground behind neck. Dig the dirt with running motion of legs, for fifteen counts. Return to original position and repeat twelve times.

Friday:

*Mountain Climber*—Position: Squatting with hands on ground, right leg drawn up to chest and left leg extended to rear with knee straight. With a fast cadence extend right foot backward and bring left leg to chest. Repeat twenty-five times.

*Wrestler's Bridge*—Position: Weight supported on toes and head. Rotate in circles to right and left.

*Leg-Back Stretch*—Position: Flat on back with arms bracing shoulders against the turn. With knee stiff, raise one leg to perpendicular position and swing it across body until foot touches hand on opposite side, shoulders flat throughout. Repeat twenty times with right, left and both legs (good for low back injuries).

*Toe and Heel Dance*—Position: One-half squatting position with trunk erect. Remaining in this position, jump to the right heel extended in front and the left toe extended behind. Jump again, reversing the order of the feet. Repeat rapidly forty times. From same position jump with the right heel to the side and left foot in place. Repeat to left.

Saturday:

*Sacro-Iliac Stretch*—Position: Sitting with knees drawn to chest. Lock arms around knees and roll back onto shoulders. Continue to roll and tighten the grip of the arms.

*Leg Stretch*—Position: Stand erect with hands at sides. Bend forward without bending knees, and touch toes. Repeat 20-30 times. Repeat same with legs crossed.

*Groin Stretcher*—Position: On knees, hands on hips, stretch backward as far as possible and return. Repeat.

*High Step-Dive*—Position: Stationary high step run-dive forward, weight on hands and let chest strike ground lightly, then abdomen, thighs and feet. Jump to feet and repeat fifteen times.

SUNDAY: *Optional*.

By September first, the athlete should be in condition to play a regulation game if it were necessary. If he watches his weight, works hard and faithfully, he will have no trouble reporting back in tip-top condition. The athlete should post the daily exercises in his bedroom.

*If Post Season Game:*

December — Practice.
January — Nothing.
February — Three times a week: Run, exercises, handball, weights, weight assignments for spring football.

*If No Post Season Game:*

December — Nothing.
January — Same as February above.
February — Step up the January program.

*March—April:*

Spring Practice — Tuesday, Wednesday, Thursday, and Saturday, for five weeks.

In addition to the above, we write to our boys throughout the summer, constantly keeping tab on those with rehabilitative and weight problems. (See Chapter 6)

Many boys need an added incentive to enable them to report in good condition. In 1948, Ivy Williamson (now Athletic Director at the University of Wisconsin) inaugurated the 6:30 mile at Lafayette College. Before the boys left for the summer they were told that each one would have to run a mile immediately following his physical examination in September. If they completed their mile in less than 6:30, they would not have to run it again. If, however, they were over 6:30, they would have to run it every day after practice until they posted their time under 6:30. Needless to say, if they did not pass their mile test the first day, it was practically impossible to pass it after a practice session. We did, however, make the boys run after every practice until a week prior to our opening game. The first year our results were good, and the following years they were much better. Many universities from time to time have used the 6:30 mile or other time standards. (Wisconsin, Illinois, Purdue, Iowa State, Miami, and the Chicago Bears)

## SUMMER CONDITIONING FOR HIGH SCHOOL ATHLETES

It is my belief that a high school athlete needs even more incentive to carry on a summer conditioning program than a college athlete. Following is a summer or off-season conditioning plan that could be inaugurated in any high school.

A. Personal letters to the boys.
B. Physical examination.
C. Start gradually, reach peak in August.
D. Give the boys a plan or chart to follow.
   1. Conditioning exercises.
   2. Run. (6:30 mile or its equivalent)
   3. Wind sprints.
   4. Step climb, forward and backward.
   5. Specific rehabilitation exercises.
   6. Temperate living.
      a. Sleep—"the great restorer"—a minimum of nine hours. Two hours before midnight is better than four after.
      b. Good Diet. (See Chapter 6)
      c. No Intoxicants. The A.M.A. has stated that "alcohol is a detriment to the human organism. Its use in therapeutics, as a tonic, food, or stimulant has no scientific value. It attacks the central nervous system. It is not a food; it is a poison."
      d. No Smoking. Nowhere is there any medical evidence that states that it improves an athlete's ability. It actually slows him up. Nicotine is a poison. If one smokes a pack of cigarettes a day for a week, he inhales 400 mg. of nicotine, which in a single injection would kill him instantly.
      e. No Drugs. The United States Olympic Committee has recently ruled that any competitor who uses

drugs, stimulants, or other substances known as "dope" for any purpose will be disqualified.

## WINNERS GIVE EVERYTHING THEY'VE GOT

Dr. Stewart Wolf, chairman of the Department of Medicine at the University of Oklahoma, recently told a group of coaches that everyone has a built in "governor" which prevents him from doing his utmost. He remarked that a big factor in winning teams is their ability to cheat on these margins and outdo them. He compared the "governor" with a regulator on a boiler, and stated that each boy has a substantial margin of safety in the "boiler," so mothers need not worry too much that their young athletes will overdo.

Coach Bud Wilkinson has often made the statement that the difference between a champion and a fellow who plays well is:

1. The fellow who slows up a little ten yards from the end of a wind sprint—this is the human trait—is lazy, takes the easy way out.

2. The champion is a man who can finish. He has no folding point.

## WEIGHT LIFTING AS PART OF THE PROGRAM

Weight lifting, like any other activity, is an ideal form of exercising if not carried to an extreme. Weight lifting alone is not recommended. It should be a part of an over-all program.

In regard to agility, muscle mass, and endurance, Dr. Robert Brashear, orthopedic surgeon of Knoxville, Tennessee, made the following comments in his booklet on *Athletic Injuries.* "Whether one is trying to rebuild a weakened muscle post-operatively, or whether one is trying to develop a boy's muscles, he must strain his muscles to the ultimate if he is to build muscle mass. We develop grace and agility by handball and boxing, by fancy diving, by the trampoline, and even by doing the jitterbug. We develop endurance by running up and down the stadium steps, but we never develop muscle mass except by strain."

A suggested weight lifting program for football players is as follows:

BUILDING STRENGTH, POWER, BODY BULK

Breathe in deeply when lifting, exhale when lowering. In the first six exercises below, start with 40 to 50 pounds and increase the weight five to ten pounds per session. Athletes should build up to maximum weight, with 15 repetitions of each exercise done in three series of five each. These exercises should be done three times a week, with adequate warm-up before each exercise period (running, stretching exercises, and rope-skipping).

1. To develop spring, initial charge, ankles, body balance and strength:
   Calf Raises—Place weight on back of neck, feet eight inches apart, body straight. Raise up on toes as high as possible.

2. To develop leg power and strength, back strength, explosive power, increase size of thoracic cage—good weight-gaining exercise.
   ¾ Knee Bends—Place weight on back of neck, feet 12 to 14 inches apart, heels flat on ground, toes pointed slightly outside, head up, shoulders back, butttocks low. Squat down to ¾ knee flexion, return to starting position. If weight is too heavy, do only a ½ squat. (Do not do a deep knee bend.)

3. To strengthen upper back muscles, pulling power, shoulder snap, fingers and wrist:
   Rowing Motion—Feet 24 to 30 inches apart, head up and forward, knees straight, but not stiff. Lift weight from ground to chest and return.

4. To strengthen lower back, shoulders, wrist and fingers:
   Stiff-Legged Dead Lifts—Bar on floor in front of feet, feet 12 to 15 inches apart, legs and arms straight. Bend at waist and grasp bar in middle of hand grip. Straighten back and lift weights up to low abdomen. Lower weights to ground in same manner as they were picked up.

5. To develop upper body, shoulders, chest, forearm, elbows, and shoulders:
   Bench Press—Lie flat on back (on bench), with feet on ground. Grasp bar on outside edge of grip of bar. Elbows

are placed wide and along line of bar. Press weights straight up, extend elbows.

6. Best all-around strength exercises. Neck, arms, back and legs:
   Place feet under bar and about 12 inches apart, toes slightly outward, head high, back and arms straight, heels down. Bend at knees and grasp bar, arms and back straight. Lift bar to low abdomen, keeping arms and back straight. Lower to ground with same body movements.

7. To build up knee and thigh:
   Quadriceps Lift—Use iron boot or table. Sit on table, knee bent. Lift foot, knee straight. Use maximum weight and lift three series of ten (30 lifts total).
   Hamstring Lift—On stomach or standing, use iron boot and raise knee to right angle. Same technique as Quadriceps Lift.

8. To build up or prevent shoulder injury:
   Bar Hang—Five chins and two minutes of hanging at arms' length.

Heavy resistance with low repetitions builds strength and high repetitions with less resistance builds endurance.

## The Ingredients of Greatness

As part of athletes' mental conditioning, the following qualities and applications can be posted in the training room.

C—oncentration
H—eart
A—ttitude
M—odesty
P—ractice
S—acrifice.

# CHAPTER IV

# Practice Routines

It is fully realized that the time spent on the practice field will vary according to such factors as the weather conditions, experience of squad, day of the week. One cannot set down any hard and fast rule, but the tendency is to practice too long, and with too much scrimmage. Many teams leave Saturday's game on the practice field. In the past eight years, we have never had a game scrimmage after the first week in October. Often we eliminate our game scrimmages before October.

Following is a chart of the time we at Oklahoma spent practicing during the 1957 and 1959 seasons:

### TIME SPENT ON PRACTICE FIELD—1957

|  | Practices | In Shorts | Avg. Time |
|---|---|---|---|
| Prior to Week of Opening Game | 23 | 5 | 1:39 |
| Week Prior to Opening Game | 6 | 5 | 1:02 |
| Week Prior to Open Date | 6 | 4 | 1:14 |
| Week Prior to Second Game | 5 | 2 | 1:07 |
| Week Prior to Third Game | 5 | 2 | 1:09 |
| Week Prior to 4th Game | 5 | 3 | 1:04 |
| Week Prior to 5th Game | 5 | 3 | 1:05 |
| Week Prior to 6th Game | 5 | 2 | :50 |
| Week Prior to 7th Game | 5 | 2 | 1:13 |
| Week Prior to 8th Game | 5 | 4 | 1:11 |
| Week Prior to 9th Game | 5 | 2 | :58 |
| Week Prior to 10th Game | 5 | 5 | :59 |
| Prior to Leaving for Orange Bowl Game | 6 | 1 | 1:13 |
| In Miami— | 8 | 4 | |

## TIME SPENT ON PRACTICE FIELD—1959

|  | *Practices* | *In Shorts* | *Avg. Time* |
|---|---|---|---|
| Prior to Week of Opening Game | 30 | 8 | 1:36 |
| Week Prior to Opening Game | 5 | 4 | 1:14 |
| Week Prior to 2nd Game | 5 | 2 | 1:31 |
| Week Prior to 3rd Game | 5 | 3 | 1:09 |
| Week Prior to 4th Game | 5 | 3 | 1:08 |
| Week Prior to 5th Game | 5 | 3 | 1:02 |
| Week Prior to 6th Game | 5 | 3 | 1:09 |
| Week Prior to 7th Game | 5 | 2 | 1:10 |
| Week Prior to 8th Game | 4 | 1 | 1:07 |
| Week Prior to 9th Game | 4 | 2 | :59 |
| Week Prior to 10th Game | 4 | 3 | :57 |

It is believed by many that a light practice routine will not work in high school. However, this has not proven to be true at Ada, Oklahoma, High School. In one of the toughest conferences in the country, Ada won six out of eight state championships and had a record of 90 victories and seven losses from 1950 through 1958.

In an article written by Ray Soldan and published in *The Daily Oklahoman* on September 18, 1955, he explains the Ada theory as follows:

The Ada Cougars, mythical state champions in 1954, are a prime example of a new theory in coaching; that you don't have to rough it up in practice to turn out a good football team.

Elvan George, Ada's veteran coach [now head coach at East Central College], limits his charges to conditioning drills, dummy scrimmages, and plenty of individual instruction. The Cougars never have game condition scrimmages and do no tackling. The only contact work the club engages in is a little hitting among the linemen.

"We don't even have practice pants," George said. "We work out in shorts all the time. The only regulation garb we wear in practices is shoulder pads and helmets and we wear those only for the feel of the equipment. Our linemen wear jerseys, but our backs just don T-shirts to keep the shoulder pads from flapping."

The highly-successful Ada pilot revealed that he has been toying with the unique practice method for three years. The club used the system 100 per cent last season for the first time and rolled triumphantly through an 11-game schedule.

The merits of the no-contact system? George cites the following:

"1. There is little chance for practice injuries. We suffered none last year.

"2. We can do considerably more running and agility work.

"3. We feel it makes our timing better.

"4. Every kid has to hustle because in our system of individual drills the coaches can see exactly what each boy is doing. In scrimmage sessions, you often see some loafing.

"5. We get an extra hour of practice a week on most teams because we work an hour and a half every Thursday. We can do it since we don't need the time to recuperate."

What are the disadvantages? "There no doubt are some," George commented, "but we're sold on our system."

In 1959, Ada won 11 and lost 2, also winning the state championship, under coach Craig McBroom. Mr. McBroom is a firm believer in Mr. George's practice policies, and he recently told me that in 1957 and 1958, when he coached at the Ada Junior High School, his teams scrimmaged only four times in the two years and they were not scored on in 1958.

During the two-a-day practice sessions at Oklahoma, we practice at 6:30 A.M. and again at 4:00 P.M. Since we do not eat breakfast until after the morning workout, we have available at the dressing room a fruit juice beverage (two parts of frozen grape juice to one part frozen lime juice). After much experimenting, it was found the boys prefer this juice to any other.

Outside the dressing room door, there is a high bar, and it is recommended that each boy hang from this bar for from one to two minutes. This is an excellent method of stretching the shoulder girdle. Prior to the opening of the practice session, the usual calisthenic routine is carried out.

During the practice sessions (before the cool weather), we take a 10-minute break midway through the afternoon session and give the boys frosted orange and lemon quarters. The boys are also given Ascorbic Acid Lozenges (Hi Score C) while on the field.

To help replenish the salt lost during practice and as an aid in quenching the boys' thirst, we make available at the dressing room door a cool saline solution for the boys to drink. In making this saline solution, we add eight to ten tablespoons of salt to 10 gal. of water. Each boy also has one cola drink after practice.

# CHAPTER V

# The Game Weekend

Our game weekend is the same whether we are playing at home or away. On Fridays we have a short practice in sweat suits (average of 20 minutes in 1957 and 17 minutes in 1959) in which we try to have the boys break a sweat and then take a refreshing shower.

At 6:00 we eat our Friday evening meal, which consists of the following:

> Fresh Fruit Cup or Large Orange Juice
> Salad (Soup in November)
> 16 oz. T-Bone Steak or Prime Rib of Beef
> Baked Potato
> Spinach and Peas
> Bread, Butter, Honey
> Tea or Pint of Milk
> Ice Cream

After dinner, the boys usually go to a movie. However, this is not compulsory. Some may rest or study at the hotel. All boys must be in their rooms by 10:00 P.M. and lights out by 10:30 P.M. Each boy is given a large apple before bed.

For a 2:00 P.M. game the squad is awakened at 8:30 A.M., and has the following meal at 9:00 A.M. (meal is not compulsory).

> Large Glass of Orange Juice
> Choice of Dry Cereal, enough Milk to moisten
> 8oz. Filet Mignon with Sauces
> Two Loosely Scrambled Eggs
> Toast, Butter, Honey
> Tea or Coffee

Following breakfast, we have a squad meeting at which time we tape all the ankles.

At 11:00 A.M. we have a pre-game lunch (not compulsory). We usually have about 15 boys who eat a part of this meal.

> Large Glass of Orange Juice
> Canned Peaches in Natural Syrup
> Toast, Butter, Honey
> Hot Tea

We leave the hotel so we will arrive at the stadium at 12:30 P.M. We then complete our taping (everything except ankles) and, if necessary, apply sun glare to the cheek bones.

*Pre-Game Nervousness*—Some boys have diet peculiarities. For example, we have had boys who cannot digest orange juice, eggs, or milk. In this event, we eliminate the food which is causing the boy's digestive problems. If it is just a pre-game nervous stomach, we have had success with Titralac, Pepto-Bismol, Kaopectate or sucking cracked ice.

*Rain Preparations*—Wear mud-cleats on which stove polish has been rubbed to keep the mud from adhering to the cleats. Assign two or three boys to go on the field at each time-out to clean the shoes. To help prevent fumbling, the boys may use any of the following on their hands: Rosin, Firm Grip, Q.D.A., Neutral Shoe Polish. To help the backs, sew a pocket in the back of their football pants in which they can keep a bag of Rosin.

*Cold Weather Preparations*—Sideline coats and blankets. Straw around players bench to keep feet warm. Rub oil of wintergreen on body before dressing. Long underwear or plastic (dry cleaning sacks) under uniform. Gloves. Chemical Heat Packs which can be held on sidelines or placed under belt on small of back—can also be taken on field at time-outs. Fire in an oil drum. Hot tea or bouillon at half-time.

*Pre-Game Equipment Preparations*—Arrange for a doctor to be on the bench and an ambulance to be at the field; stretchers, oxygen, ice packs, necessary medications and protective equipment.

*Preparations for Visiting Team*—Provide a manager to run errands; a training table in a well-lighted room; a stretcher on their bench; medical care if they do not have a physician with them; instructions on where the ambulance is located; towels, water, chewing gum; equipment that they may have forgotten; and cola drinks or fruit as they desire.

*Care of Boys on Sidelines and at Time-Outs*—Trainer should watch the field at all time. If for any reason he has to take his eyes off the field, he should assign one of his assistants to watch and to call him immediately if there is an injury. Watch every play as this can give a definite clue as to what type of injury to expect. Assign one assistant to sponge off and check for injuries all boys coming out of the game, and one assistant to provide them with water and ascorbic acid lozenges. At time-outs assign one assistant to take water (in a plastic squirt-bottle) and towels on the field. The trainer should also go on the field to check injuries, fatigue, and to give the boys smelling salts and oil of peppermint.

*Half-Time Procedures*—Check all injuries while the assistants check equipment and provide the boys with oranges, cola drinks, Dextrose B$^1$ tablets, oxygen, ice bags, or chewing gum. In cold weather, we also have hot sweetened tea available. We do not tell the boys how much to eat or drink at the half. We leave that up to them.

Following the game, when we are away from home, we have sandwiches, milk, and cola drinks in the dressing room. As soon as the boys reach the plane, we have available as much orange juice as they wish. Our meal on the plane usually consists of the following:

> Fruit Cup
> Salad
> ½ Fried Chicken
> Mashed Potatoes
> Vegetables
> Roll, Butter
> Ice Cream (all they want)
> Milk (all they want)

Following home games, we have cola drinks in the dressing room and after the boys are dressed they go to our training table where they have a meal similar to the one described above (on plane).

*Sunday Morning Routine*—Our training room is open from 9:00 A.M. to 11:00 A.M. and every boy who played on Saturday is to report for a steam bath or a treatment if injured. We require all boys to take a six- to ten-minute steam bath to eliminate the soreness from Saturday's game.

*CHAPTER VI*

# The Athlete's Diet

A wholesome diet for an athlete should be composed of a variety of good foods. There is no magic pill, wonder food, or sure-fire formula which will make one a better athlete, but a proper diet will help to keep one at his best. To help select a variety of foods, I can think of no better method than by using the *FOODWAY to FOLLOW* plan.

One should start every day with a good, solid, substantial breakfast (fruit or fruit juice, cereal, eggs, ham or bacon, toast and beverage). Breakfast is the foundation for the day, and no building or day is any better than its foundation. The breakfast is without a doubt the most important meal of the day, and should include at least 1/3 of the daily caloric intake. Although this fact was known for years, the Navy recently proved it without question. Trying to find an explanation for many unexplained air accidents, it was found that the pilots involved had eaten inadequate or no breakfast at all. Navy pilots were then required to eat a good, solid breakfast and a reduction in the unexplained accidents was observed immediately. It is now known that many accidents can be blamed on slowed reaction resulting from insufficient food sugar for the brain to function at top efficiency.

DIET FACTS

Food you eat today takes 36 hours before it is in the system in the form of weight. Your weight today increased or decreased according to what you ate 36 hours ago.

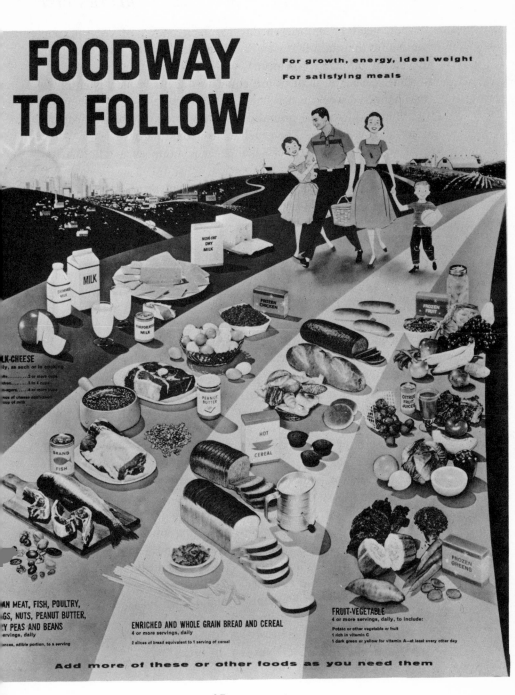

37

You need 15 calories a day for each pound of your present weight, to maintain that weight. By adding 1000 a day, you gain. By taking off 1000 (or more), you lose.

One thousand calories are equal to 4.2 ozs, which is equal to two pounds a week.

After reducing 20 pounds, it is like being on the 4-yard line after a 20-yard run. The touchdown is the toughest.

Two pieces of fried chicken are the same as a whole roast chicken.

A high protein diet is satisfactory—lean meat and fish (not fried), eggs (boiled or poached), cheese, skimmed milk.

It is hard to gain weight on any vegetable. Many dietitians say it is impossible.

Fat will not gather around a working muscle. The tummy and rear of fat boys harbor the most fat. To reduce the tummy, try walking to the bathroom and back on all fours. You have never seen a four-legged animal with a bay window. To reduce the seat area, try wiggling in synchronization with your toothbrush as you slide the brush back and forth across the molars.

Do not eat yourself out of the league. It takes will power and work to reduce.

A sandwich has more calories than a filet. A double-decker sandwich usually has more calories than a vegetable plate plus dessert.

Twelve cups of consomme are equal to one large bowl of cream of tomato soup.

Two glasses of water weigh approximately one pound.

You lose one to two pounds in a night's sleep.

An overweight person expends more energy and burns more of his body reserve to accomplish the same amount of work than he would if he were at recommended weight.

The meal prior to an athletic contest should be eaten three to four hours before the contest.

Salt should be supplemented in the diet during hot weather conditions and during profuse sweating.

An athlete should eat three good meals a day, the most important being breakfast. Never skip breakfast.

## JEFFERSON TRAINING TABLE — MENUS FOR
## FIRST WEEK IN NOVEMBER

### MONDAY

| *Breakfast* | *Lunch* | *Dinner* |
|---|---|---|
| Juice or Prunes | Country Special | Roast Beef with |
| Cereals | Pinto Beans |    Brown Gravy |
| Bacon & Eggs | Spiced Ham | Snow Flake Potatoes |
| Toast & Jelly | Spinach, | Frozen |
| Milk & Coffee |    Sliced Tomatoes |    Mixed Vegetables |
| | Sliced Onions | Lettuce Wedges with |
| | Hot Corn Bread, |    Thousand Island |
| |    Peaches |    Dressing |
| | Tea (Iced or Hot) | Fruit Cobbler |
| | | Iced Tea & Milk |

### TUESDAY

| | | |
|---|---|---|
| Juice or Fruit | Vegetable Soup with | Grilled T-Bone Steaks |
| Sweet Rolls (Hot) |    Crackers | Baked Potatoes with |
| Eggs | Bacon & Tomato |    Butter |
| Cereals |    Sandwiches | Peas |
| Toast & Jelly | Shredded Lettuce & | Tossed Salad |
| Milk & Coffee |    Cottage Cheese | Mixed Fruit and |
| |    with Fruit |    Oatmeal Cookies |
| | Ice Cream or Fruit | Tea & Milk |
| | Tea (Iced or Hot), | |
| |    Lemonade | |

### WEDNESDAY

| | | |
|---|---|---|
| Juice or Fruit | Tomato Soup or Broth | Cured Ham Baked |
| Cereals |    with Crackers |    or Beef Roast |
| Cured Ham | Creamed Chicken on | Green Beans |
| Eggs |    Toast or Beef | Waldorf Salad |
| Toast & Jelly | Lettuce & Egg Salad | Chocolate Cake |
| Milk & Coffee |    with Dressing | Milk & Iced Tea |
| | Fruited Jellos | |
| | Iced Tea | |

### THURSDAY

| | | |
|---|---|---|
| Juice or Prunes | Beef Soup or Potato | Breaded Steaks & |
| Hot Cakes & Bacon |    Soup with Crackers |    Cream Gravy |
| Syrup | Three varieties of | Mashed Potatoes |
| Cereals |    Meat & | Peas or Buttered Beets |
| Toast & Jelly |    Toasted Sandwiches | Lettuce Wedges with |
| Milk & Coffee |    (Cheese) |    Thousand Island |
| | Tomatoes on Lettuce |    Dressing |
| | Baked Apples | Peaches or Pears |
| | Tea (Iced or Hot), | Tea & Milk |
| |    Lemonade | |

FRIDAY

| | | |
|---|---|---|
| Cereal | Fresh Catfish with | Beef Roast with |
| Cheese Omelet | Tartar Sauce | Brown Gravy or |
| Juice or Fruit | or Beef Roast | Smothered Liver |
| Cinnamon Toast | Macaroni & Cheese | Buttered Potatoes |
| Toast & Jelly | Cabbage Slaw | Combination Salad |
| Milk & Coffee | Lettuce | Cherry Pudding |
| | Lemon Pudding or | Milk & Tea |
| | Fruit | |
| | Tea (Iced or Hot) | |

SATURDAY

| | | |
|---|---|---|
| Juice or Fruit | Hot Beef Sandwiches | Sliced Ham, |
| Scrambled Eggs & | Mashed Potatoes | Cold Sliced Turkey |
| Sausage | Green Beans | Baked Beans or |
| Cereals | Variety Salads | Potato Salad |
| Donuts | Ice Cream | Sliced Tomatoes or |
| Toast & Jelly | Tea (Iced or Hot) | Lettuce Leaves |
| Milk & Coffee | | Cake & Lemonade |
| | | Tea & Milk |
| | | (If weather cold, Hot Soup) |

SUNDAY

| | | |
|---|---|---|
| Juice or Fruit | Fried Chicken & | Bread & Butter each |
| Donuts | Cream Gravy | meal (no limit). |
| Eggs & Cereal | Snowflake Potatoes | Typical weekly |
| Toast & Jelly | Frozen Peas | menu. Only change |
| Milk & Coffee | Combination Salad | would be meat, |
| | Hot Rolls & Honey | salad & beverages. |
| | Strawberry Shortcake | Roast beef available |
| | with Whipped Cream | every lunch and |
| | Tea or Milk | dinner if athlete (in season) does not like meat that is being served. |

## SUGGESTIONS FOR LOSING WEIGHT

Reduce only under medical supervision.

Do not skip meals.

Eat a large breakfast, a moderate lunch, and a light dinner. Food eaten at breakfast is absorbed by the body during the day and is not stored as fat as with the evening meal.

Eat nothing between meals or before bedtime.

Continue with daily activity—exercise.

Use saccharine (no caloric value) instead of sugar.

Do not drink large amounts of water with meals. Try to hold

the fluid intake to not more than one quart per day (average is eight glasses).

Use a minimum of salt. It helps retain water.

Weigh yourself at the same time each day, preferably upon arising.

Eat high protein foods, vegetables, and salads.

Substitute lemon juice or vinegar for salad dressings.

There is only one miracle drug—sulpha-denial.

### BEWARE OF THE FOLLOWING

|  | *Amount* | *Calories* |
|---|---|---|
| Chocolate malt | 8 oz. | 400 |
| Chocolate milk | 8 oz. | 350 |
| Cocoa | 8 oz. | 300 |
| Carbonated beverage | 6 oz. | 85 |
| Lemonade | 8 oz. | 175 |
| Sweet roll | small | 135 |
| Corn bread | 2 in. sq. | 140 |
| French toast | 1 | 130 |
| White bread | 1 | 70 |
| Saltine crackers | each | 30 |
| Oatmeal | 8 oz. | 200 |
| Grape nuts | 8 oz. | 400 |
| Donuts | 1 | 200-350 |
| Wheat cakes | small | 125 |
| Spaghetti (plain) | ¾ cup | 110 |
| Baked apple | 1 | 210 |
| Fruit cocktail | ½ cup | 100 |
| Stewed prunes | 4 | 170 |
| Banana | small | 100 |
| Peanuts | 8 | 90 |
| Pecans | 6 | 115 |
| Walnuts | 8 | 190 |
| Brazil nuts | 4 | 200 |
| Cashews | 8 small | 90 |
| French dressing | tbs. | 75 |
| Mayonnaise | tbs. | 95 |
| Thousand Island dressing | tbs. | 100 |
| Corn oil | tbs. | 100 |
| Bean soup | 8 oz. | 200 |
| Cream soups | 8 oz. | 200 |
| Iced cake | 2½ in. sq. | 300 |
| Fruit pie | 1/6 cut | 350 |

## BEWARE OF THE FOLLOWING

|  | *Amount* | *Calories* |
|---|---|---|
| Cream pie | 1/6 cut | 400 |
| Strawberry shortcake | average | 450 |
| Oatmeal cookie | 3½″ diam. | 120 |
| Baked custard | ⅝ cup | 185 |
| Chocolate sundae | 6 oz. | 400 |
| Chocolate ice cream soda | Fountain | 400 |
| Vanilla ice cream | 1/6 qt. | 200 |
| Chocolate ice cream | 1/6 qt. | 280 |
| Strawberry sundae | 6 oz. | 450 |
| Baked beans | ½ cup | 120 |
| Corn on cob | med. | 100 |
| Mashed potatoes | ½ cup | 155 |
| Sweet candied potato | med. | 275 |
| French fried potato | each | 20 |
| Butter | tbs. | 100 |
| Peanut butter | tbs. | 100 |
| Popcorn | 1 cup | 55 |
| Candy bar | 2 oz. | 275 |
| Crackerjack | Box | 250 |
| Peanut bar | small | 350 |
| Catsup | tbs. | 25 |
| Honey, jam, jelly | tbs. | 60 |
| Potato chips | each | 10 |
| Pretzels | small, each | 10 |
| Hamburger sandwich | small | 400 |
| Ham and cheese sandwich | one | 450 |
| Hot dog sandwich | small | 300 |

## SAMPLE OF AN APPROXIMATE 1000-CALORIE DIET

(Do not diet without doctor's permission).

BREAKFAST

| | |
|---|---|
| Tomato Juice, ½ cup | 25 calories |
| Corn Flakes, 1 cup | 80 |
| Skim Milk to moisten | 20 |
| 2 Eggs, Boiled or Poached | 140 |
| 1 Strip Crisp Bacon, 4 x 1 in. | 30 |
| Bread, 1 slice | 70 |
| Tea or Coffee, Black | 00 |
| | —— |
| | 365 |

(same as a Piece of Pie)

LUNCH

|  |  |
|---|---|
| Hamburger Patty, lean, 1/5 lb. | 140 calories |
| Green Beans, canned, ½ cup | 20 |
| Cantaloupe, ½ | 40 |
| Skimmed Milk, 8 oz. | 85 |
| Bread, 1 slice | 70 |
| (same as 8 oz. Chocolate Milk) | 355 |

DINNER

|  |  |
|---|---|
| Veal Cutlet (average) | 100 |
| Tomatoes, ½ cup (canned or medium fresh) | 20 |
| Mixed Green Salad, light oil | 30 |
| Grapefruit, ½ | 45 |
| Skimmed Milk, 8 oz. | 85 |
| Bread, ½ slice | 35 |
| (same as a Hot Dog) | 315 |

## TWO-WEEK REDUCING DIET

(Do not diet without doctor's permission).

This diet is based on chemical reaction and maintenance of normal energy while reducing. Unless specified, eat as much as you wish. Weight should decrease about 18-20 lbs. in two weeks.

Diet is for only two weeks. Eat everything assigned and nothing else. Do not eat between meals.

No fried foods or salads with oil, no butter, eat lean meat, coffee black, tea clear.

Breakfast—Same every day: Grapefruit, 1 or 2 eggs, ½ slice dry toast, coffee or tea.

MONDAY

*Lunch*—2 eggs, grapefruit, coffee or tea.
*Dinner*—steak, tomatoes, lettuce, celery, cucumbers, olives, coffee
    or tea.

TUESDAY

*Lunch*—2 eggs, spinach, tomatoes, coffee or tea.
*Dinner*—2 lamb chops or equivalent in roast beef, tomatoes, cu-
    cumbers, celery, coffee or tea.

WEDNESDAY

*Lunch*—2 eggs, spinach, coffee or tea.
*Dinner*—cold chicken, tomatoes, grapefruit, coffee or tea.

THURSDAY

*Lunch*—2 eggs, spinach, coffee or tea.
*Dinner*—plenty of steak, tomatoes, cucumbers, celery, coffee or tea.

FRIDAY

*Lunch*—2 eggs, tomatoes, coffee or tea.
*Dinner*—2 eggs, combination salad, grapefruit, coffee or tea.

SATURDAY

*Lunch*—big fruit salad, coffee or tea.
*Dinner*—plenty of steak, tomatoes, cucumbers, celery, coffee, tea or milk.

SUNDAY

*Lunch*—2 eggs, cottage cheese, cabbage, coffee or tea.
*Dinner*—chicken, cooked cabbage, carrots, grapefruit, coffee or tea.

## SUGGESTIONS FOR GAINING WEIGHT

1. Physical examination.
2. Avoid undue fatigue, take moderate exercise, relax.
3. Eat high-calorie food slowly and often—
   mid-morning, mid-afternoon and before-bed lunches.
4. More sleep and mid-afternoon naps.
5. Reverse procedure listed under "Suggestions for Losing Weight".

## PRE-COMPETITION MEALS

There are many theories as to what an athlete should eat, pre-game meal or otherwise. I do not feel anyone should dictate to any individual what he should eat, and even whether he should eat. A dedicated athlete can usually be relied upon to use good judgment in general training habits. We have had many great athletes who have contributed outstanding performances on diets many believe an individual should not compete on. As examples, I recall a great high school basketball player who had a hamburger for breakfast and scored in the neighborhood of 40 points in a tournament game that noon; and one of our great milers who ran a truly great race in the Philadelphia Inquirer Relays shortly after eating fried chicken and French fried potatoes. Fortunately, most athletes like steak, roast beef or eggs, thus minimizing the problem of pre-game meals.

Herb Elliott, great miler from Australia, has for a training diet oats, nuts, raisins, dried fruits, and diced bananas.

The Russian wrestling team, when they toured the United States, had the following pre-match meal at our training table: 12 oz. steak, peas, baked potato, toast, honey, fruit salad, ice cream, and tea.

Bill Nieder, first man to put the 16-lb. shot 65 feet had the following meal prior to his historic throw (65' 7"): 7:00 A.M.— extra large steak, three eggs, three strips of bacon, two large glasses of orange juice, half pint of milk. At 10:00 A.M. he had a second large steak and a piece of pie.

J. D. Martin, Oklahoma's fine pole vaulter, prefers a small rare steak, toast, honey, and hot tea about three and one-half hours before competing.

The Finnish Olympic Cross-Country Skiing Team, following a normal breakfast, drinks large quantities of eggnog (with a half dozen or more raw eggs) prior to starting on the cross country event. Along the course, they have "snack stations" where the racers pause long enough to pick up a cup of quick energy. The Finns' quick-energy concoction is Mustikakeito, which consists of blueberries, heated in water with sugar added. Other quick-energy drinks on the ski course were lukewarm, sugared water, with or without honey. Other preparations for quick energy are:

Dextrose tablets; honey; two tablespoons of honey to eight ounces or orange juice; glass of water flavored with lemon or orange to which is added as much dextrose or honey as liked and a half teaspoon of salt; to one pint of tea add six tablespoons of honey and orange juice to suit taste, serve cool, not cold.

Oklahoma football pre-game meals are listed in Chapter V and basketball in Chapter XX.

# CHAPTER VII

# Types of Injuries and
# Their General Treatment

In diagnosing an injury, one should take into consideration:

1. What one sees.
2. What one hears.
3. What one feels.
4. Answers to questions (history).
5. Comparison—deformity?
6. Reason and common sense.

## Types of Injuries

1. Bone Fractures—divided into a number of types depending on the nature of the break. Some of the most common are:

   1. *Greenstick*—bone is cracked and bent, but not completely broken off. Usually found in children and may be compared to a break in a green twig when sharply bent.
   2. *Simple*—bone is broken, but not the skin.
   3. *Compound*—bone and skin are broken, bone protrudes through the skin.
   4. *Comminuted*—a splintering of the bone at the site of the fracture, crushed.
   5. *Impacted*—telescoping of the ends of the bone has taken place.

6. *Multiple*—bone broken in more than one place.

7. *Oblique* (spiral)—break extends diagonally across the bone.

8. *Transverse*—break extends across the bone, at right angles to its long axis.

*Recognition*

1. Boy may have heard a "click."
2. Tenderness and swelling at point of injury.
3. Crepitus or grating of the bone.
4. Sudden stabbing pain on movement.
5. Muscles in area may contract.
6. Deformity.
7. Sick at stomach. (Shock—Chapter XVI)

2. Nerve

*Recognition*

Burning sensation—like being hit on the "crazy bone" —numb, pins, needles.

3. Muscle
4. Tendon
5. Ligament
6. Joint

Worse on movement, dull pain, may be over an elongated area, stiffen up overnight. Ligament and tendon injuries— loose joint can be compared to opposite joint.

Effusion—fills up with fluid. If so, boy may say his joint feels as though it is being gripped hard by a number of moving fingers.

7. Compensation—is in reality a false injury. Often called a cause and effect injury. A boy is injured in a specific area, and to relieve the pain in this area, he throws an undue strain on another area of the body. Before long, he feels as if he had been injured in the second area.

CLASSIFICATION OF INJURIES

1. Contusion (Above # 1, 2, 3, 4, 5, 6).

A severe bruise with rupture of capillaries (hematoma), nerves and involved tissue.

2. Strain (Above # 2, 3, 4, 5, 6).

Injury to muscular and tendinous tissue—capillaries and nerves.

3. Sprain (Above # 4, 5, 6).

Injury to ligamentous tissue—capillaries, nerves, bursae, capsule, etc.

### Severity of Injury

1. Mild—fibers pulled apart, separated. Very little loss of function.

2. Moderate—fibers partially torn. Some loss of function.

3. Severe—fibers completely torn. Complete loss of function.

In all of the above injuries, capillaries are torn. The blood will follow the capillary groove until the capillary is restored. An example of a torn capillary: if one slaps his arm hard, it will immediately turn red. This is blood from the broken capillaries.

### Control Hemorrhage

I.  Convalescent period will be greatly reduced.

II. Will reduce fibrous scarring of tissue.

A.  Pressure (to reduce flow of blood and lymph along with ice and elevation).

1. Felt or sponge pad over area.
2. Wrap with a wet elastic bandage, extend at least 6″ above and below injury.

B. Ice

1. A minimum of 45 minutes to an hour. Continue for 24-48 hours if swelling persists.
2. Dr. E. T. Smith, Houston, Texas says the advantages of cold are:

(a) Alleviate pain and make the boy feel better.

(b) By reducing the temperature of a cell, the metabolism of the cell is reduced and given a chance to come back again, like a runner who runs a mile, rests, and can then run again.

    C. Elevation.

    D. Heat.

        1. Be careful as heat will cause swelling.

        2. If the area throbs or swells, the heat is too hot.

## GENERAL TREATMENT—CONTUSION, STRAIN, SPRAIN

Same as controlling hemorrhage—pressure, ice, elevation.

## RECOVERY TIME

Dr. M. M. Novich, Newark, N. J., lists recovery time as follows:

    I. Fractures

        A. Toes, fingers—two to three weeks.

        B. Elbow—activity resumed after ten days to eliminate the tendency of adhesions.

        C. Major bone—minimum of six weeks.

    II. Contusion, Strains—two to 21 days.

    III. Sprains—seven to 21 days.

    IV. Dislocations.

        A. Major joint—four weeks.

        B. Finger, toe—after acute symptoms subside.

## GENERAL RULES—TREATMENT

    I. Immediate

        A. Elevation, if possible.

        B. Ultra-sound. Use own judgment.

        C. Wet pressure bandage, if possible.

        D. Ice, minimum 45 minutes.

        E. If no swelling:

            1. Light Cramergesic pack with support, or

            2. Support only.

        F. If swelling—Support plus ice (no heat).

        G. *If in doubt, refer to team physician.*

    II. Second Day

        A. If swelling is severe:

            1. Pressure bandage, ice, elevation and support.

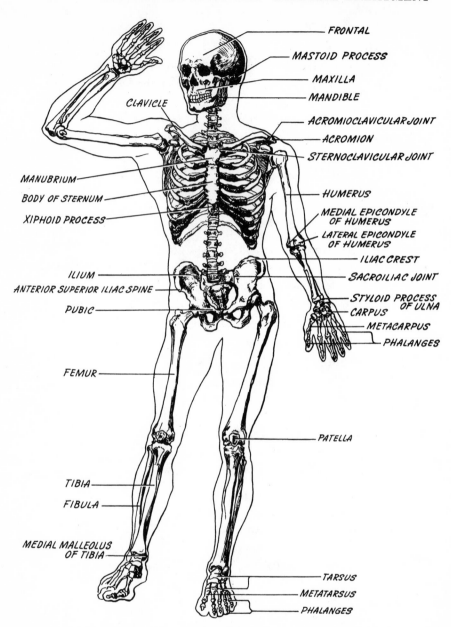

Diagram A. The Human Skeleton* (front view).

*Diagrams A and B supplied with compliments of Cramer Chemical Co., Gardner, Kansas.

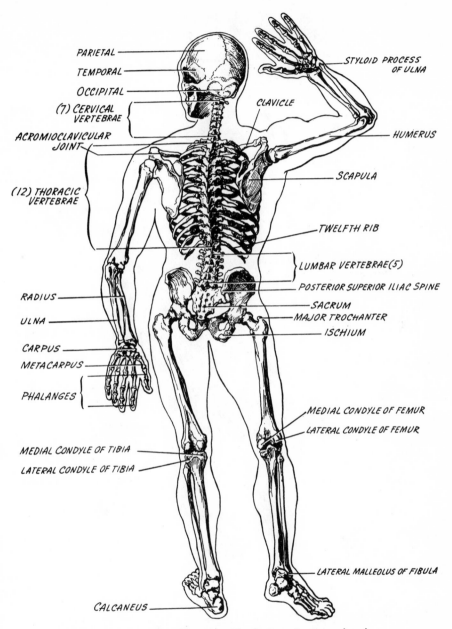

Diagram B. The Human Skeleton (rear view).

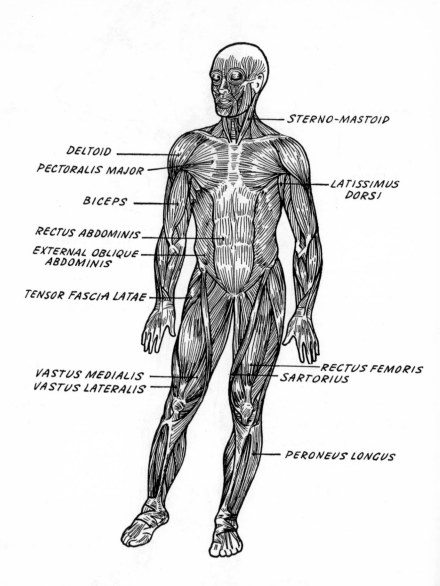

Diagram C. Muscles of the Body (front view).

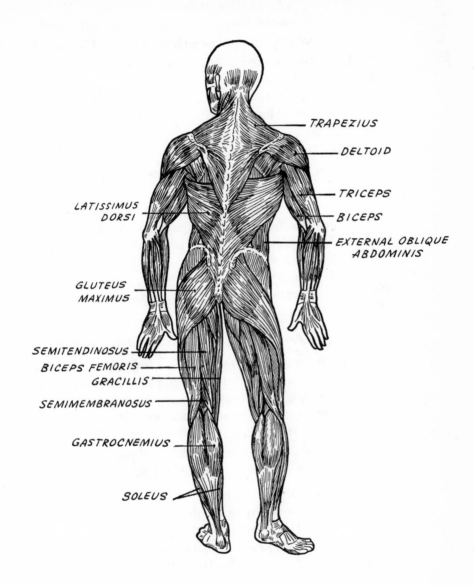

Diagram **D.** Muscles of the Body (rear view).

B. If no swelling, or light swelling:
1. Infra-red lamp—with or without wet towel
2. Whirlpool (follow whirlpool rules—Chapter II)
C. Light massage above and below injury.
D. Ultra-sound.
E. Contrast baths.
F. Cramergesic Packs.
G. Support.

III. Third Day

If swelling, follow swelling rules; if not:
1. Any of the above.
2. Microtherm, only after 48 hours, especially in any injury (joints, etc.) where there is a chance of swelling.
3. Hydrocollator steam packs.
4. Medcollator.
5. Massage.
6. Rehabilatative exercises, if possible.
7. Support, if necessary.

*Heat may cause excessive swelling—cold reduces swelling*

Alleviate fear, minimize injuries. If an individual is in shock, everything that is said will make a definite impression on him. If he is not in shock, do not say or do anything that will put him there. When in shock, the mind is wide open for suggestion and anything said will stick there.

As in all phases of athletics, the follow-through is important in the treatment of injuries, day or night if necessary.

1. Don't *Preach*.
2. Don't *Probe* too deeply.
3. Don't *Promise* too much.
4. Don't *Punish* with lectures.
5. No *Platitudes* (trite utterances).

Following on the next immediate pages are diagrams showing the skeletal and muscular structure of the body. A knowledge of the names and locations of these parts is most essential and helpful in treating athletic injuries. DIAGRAMS A, B, C, D.

# CHAPTER VIII

# Taping and Bandaging, Treating Skin Injuries, Stopping Bleeding

### TEARING TAPE (FIGURE 1.)

1. Hands should be free of surface oil.
2. Backing of the tape should face the trainer.
3. Firmly grasp the tape with thumbs held closely to each other, and index fingers directly below the thumbs. Tape must be taut.

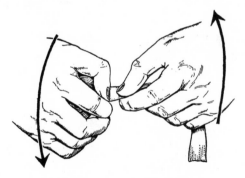

FIGURE 1. Tearing Tape.

4. Make a quick snap of the right wrist away from the body, and at the same time rotate the left wrist toward the body. Some will resist with the left wrist.
5. The secret is in breaking the first thread.

6. If not successful in tearing the tape in the first attempt, do not try again in the same place.

## RULES FOR TAPING

1. Skin preparation—wash, shave and apply Tuf Skin.
2. Use the size of tape which fits the contour of the body.
3. Have injured area in the position in which it is to remain.
4. Tape from the roll. Do not squeeze.
5. Apply smoothly, mold.
6. Strap firmly, avoid constriction and circular taping.
7. For support tape directly on the skin.
8. Basketweave tape for additional strength at stress points.

If an individual is allergic to adhesive tape, try changing brands or taping over Q.D.A., Ace Adherent, Resi Film, or Stockinett. If a rash develops, use Calamine Lotion, Ivy Dry or Nitrotan.

## RULES FOR APPLYING BANDAGE

1. Be neat, clean and thorough.
2. Use simplest application.
3. Have injured area in the position it is to remain.
4. Anchor bandage so it will not slip (tape on start, or bandage on an angle).
5. Start at narrowest part of the limb and bandage toward the heart.
6. Bandage firmly, but avoid constriction. Invert or evert (twist) the bandage.

## ABRASIONS

Abrasions are rubbing off of the skin by mechanical means; floor burn, strawberry, cinder burn.

*Treatment:*
1. Wash thoroughly with athletic liquid soap.
2. If debris (cinders) in wound, use sterile forceps to remove.
3. Irrigate with Hydrogen Peroxide.
4. Apply Nitrotan compress for several hours (gauze pad saturated with Nitrotan).

5.  Apply Zinc Oxide, Strawberry Ointment or Spectrocin and cover with a Telfa pad which will not stick to the wound.

6.  Do not permit a scab to form.

## LACERATION

Skin and tissue is torn with more or less jagged edges.

*Treatment:*

1.  Same treatment as for abrasions except wash the laceration lengthwise of the cut.

2.  Refer to physician, suturing may be necessary.

## INCISED WOUND

A straight-edged wound (a "cut").

*Treatment:*

1.  Follow first three phases of treatment for abrasions.

2.  Apply Merthiolate or Nitrotan.

3.  If necessary, hold together with a Butterfly closure (Figure 2)—purchase from Johnson and Johnson or make your own.

4.  Refer to physician, suturing may be necessary.

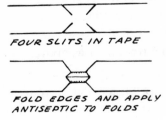

FOUR SLITS IN TAPE

FOLD EDGES AND APPLY
ANTISEPTIC TO FOLDS

FIGURE 2. Slitting tape.

## PUNCTURE WOUND

Deep piercing wound (nail, spike).

*Treatment:*

1.  Thorough washing and cleaning out of any foreign matter.

2.  Soak punctured area in a warm aseptic solution to keep it open.

3.  Encourage bleeding.

4.  Send to physician for probable tetanus shot. Bacitracin, Spectrocin.

**BLISTERS**

Blisters are due to friction.

*Treatment:*

A.  Filled with fluid.

1.  Wash blister and surrounding area with alcohol or Iso-Quin.
2.  Open at back edge (¼ in. slit) with a sterile scalpel—knife (Figure 3).

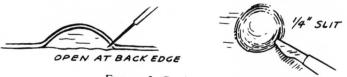

OPEN AT BACK EDGE          ¼" SLIT

FIGURE 3. Cutting a blister.

3.  Fill with antiseptic. Merthiolate, Nitrotan.
4.  Apply Zinc Oxide or Strawberry Ointment to a sterile gauze pad and cover.
5.  After blister has healed (2nd or 3rd day), trim away the loose skin. Bevel the edges.
6.  File or sandpaper the rough, loose edges of the skin and paint with Tuf Skin.

B.  Broken open—same treatment as above.

C.  Infected.

1.  Thoroughly clean blister and surrounding area (alcohol, Iso-Quin) and trim away all blistered skin and loose edges.
2.  Soak the foot in an alcohol and boric acid solution or in a boric acid solution.
3.  Apply a wet dressing (Chapter XVI), Bacitracin, Spectrocin.
4.  See team physician.

D.  Protection while playing.

1.  Cover blister with sterile dressing and cover with:

a.  Felt doughnut. Take a piece of ⅜″ felt and cut a hole in it, little larger than size of blister. Tape to hold in place.
b.  Spoon. Cut the handle off a spoon. Shape the

spoon to suit the situation and tape over blister. Inner and side edges of spoon can be covered with thin layer of moleskin (Figure 6).

2. Cover blister with collodion.

CONTROL OF BLEEDING

ARTERY—characterized by a profuse flow of bright red blood. May be in spurts.

VEIN—characterized by steady flow of dark red blood which may be of considerable volume but does not come in spurts.

CAPILLARY—characterized by a steady ooze. Is not serious and is easily controlled.

*Treatment:*

1. Hand pressure—direct pressure on the wound by hand over a sterile gauze pad.

2. Pressure bandage—roller bandage or a half dozen gauze pads tied firmly over the sterile gauze compress.

3. Pressure points—in the more complicated and severe forms of bleeding (artery), apply pressure at a point where the artery is relatively near the surface and close to a bony structure. Enclosed chart illustrates the pressure points where arterial bleeding may be reached and checked (Figure 4).

4. Tourniquet—last and least practical type of pressure. It was formerly taught that a tourniquet should not be left on for over 15 to 20 minutes. However, some physicians now believe it should be left in place until loosened by a physician (Figure 4).

5. Normal venous or capillary bleeding:
   (a) Nitrotan compress, Hydrogen Peroxide or Adrenalin Chloride 1:1000.
   (b) Doctor's recommendations: Gelfoam, Hemo Pak.

*Closing Wounds:*

1. Bandage—paint surrounding area with Q.D.A. or Ace Adherent and dressing will hold longer. Use elastic tape as it will adhere better.

2. Butterfly (Figure 2).

3. Collodion.

4. Suturing by physician.

# COMPRESSION TO CHECK ARTERIAL BLEEDING

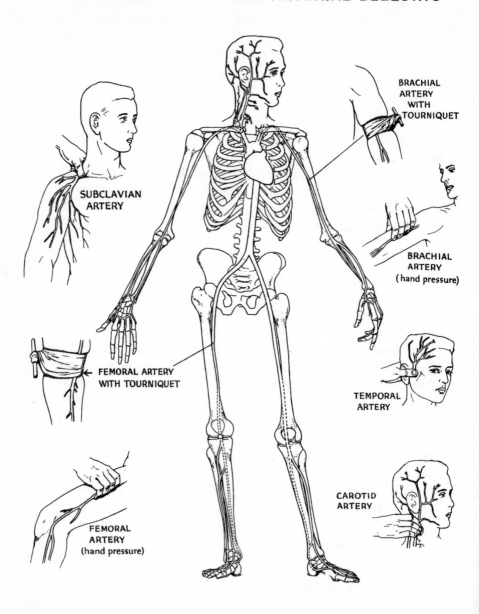

FIGURE 4. Courtesy of Cramer Chemical Co., Gardner, Kansas.

# INTRODUCTION TO CHAPTER IX THROUGH CHAPTER XVI

*Many excellent drugs, medications, ointments, etc. are now on the market. In the following chapters, I will mention what our doctors are using along these lines at the present time. In years to come, as medical science discovers better medications, the trainer must keep abreast of the time and work hand in hand with his team physician to insure athletes the very best and most modern treatment.*

*In the following chapters, I will not go into detailed treatments of the various injuries as this has been discussed in Chapter 7.*

# CHAPTER IX

# Foot and Ankle Care

### PROTECTION OF THE FEET

Condition the feet before the season starts by applying Tuf Skin twice per day. While the Tuf Skin is still "tacky," apply powder to the feet. Continue to use the Tuf Skin and powder after the season has started. You may also wish to wear two pair of socks, and if the inner seam of the shoe is bothersome, try rubbing soap on the seam.

### HOT SPOTS

*Recognition*—A burning hot sensation on the bottom of the foot. No fluid.

*Treatment*—Soak the foot in cold water for ten minutes. Rub a small amount of a bland ointment into the hot spot before the next practice.

### BRUISED OR BROKEN TOE

*Recognition*—Deformity, pain, tenderness, swelling.

*Treatment*—Immediately soak in cold water for a minimum of 45 minutes. Starting the second day, use whirlpool or soak in warm Epsom Salt solution.

*Taping*—Immobilize by taping the injured toe to the adjoining toe or toes, or place a collodion cast (gauze and collodion).

*Protective Equipment*—As soon as the soreness is gone, cut the toe out of an old shoe and make a hard protective covering out of fiber glass, castex or galvanized tin (Figure 6), to shield the injury. Tape the protective covering to the shoe. See Sprained Big Toe.

### SPRAINED BIG TOE

*Recognition and Treatment*—Same as for a bruised or broken toe.

*Taping*—Immobilize the joint. Secure a ⅜ inch felt pad to the foot (Figure 5).

*Protective Equipment*—Same as for a bruised or broken toe. Also one can tape a small block of wood under the street shoe just behind the big toe joint (Figure 5). This will permit natural walking and will hasten recovery.

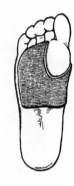

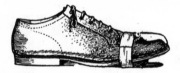

FIGURE 5. Taping sprained toe, with supported shoe.

### BLOOD UNDER TOE NAIL

*Treatment*—Remove the blood by drilling through toe-nail with the end of a knife or nail drill (Figure 6). Treat as an open wound.

*Protection*—Same as for a bruised or broken toe.

### INGROWN TOE NAIL

*Recognition*—Inflamed and swollen area along the medial or lateral sides of the big toe nail. Toe nail has grown down into the skin.

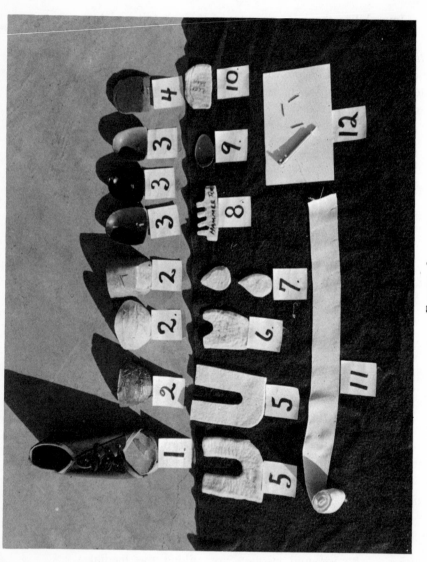

FIGURE 6.

1. Orthopedic Shoe
2. Toe Protectors (fiberglass, castex, tin)
3. Heel Protectors
4. Sponge Heel Pad
5. Felt "U"
6. Protection for Big Toe Joint
7. Transverse arch pads
8. Hammer Toe Pads
9. Spoon
10. Longitudinal Arch Pad
11. Ankle Wrap
12. Nail Drill

*Prevention*—Wear proper fitting shoes and cut the nail *straight* across, not shorter than the flesh.

*Treatment*—Cut a "V" in the top of the nail, shave the nail (very thin from the bottom of the "V" down to the base of the cuticle. Soak in Epsom Salts. Soak a small piece of cotton in alcohol, Nitrotan or Ichthammol and force under the edges of the nail. This will lift and force the nail to grow properly. Cover with collodion or a bandage.

## ATHLETE'S FOOT

*Recognition*—A reddened, irritated area with or without blisters. Caused by a fungus or plant parasite.

*Prevention*—Keep the area dry at all times; foot powder; wear white cotton socks; do not wear rubber-soled shoes.

*Treatment*—Dry thoroughly (don't rub harshly) between the toes at all times and use foot powder in shoes.

1. No blister—most common. Spreads with perspiration; can be found anywhere on body. Treat with ultra-violet light, sun, foot powder, Mycozol, Desenex, Fungo Spray, Potassium Permanganate, Sopronol.

2. Blister type. Open and soak in Potassium Permanganate one hour two times a day. Use ultra-violet light or sun and follow with one of the above ointments or liquids.

*Doctor's Recommendation*—Griseo Fulvin.

## FOOT ODORS AND PERSPIRING FEET

*Treatment*—Change the socks and shoes daily; do not wear rubber-soled shoes or nylon socks; wash feet thoroughly three times a day; soak feet in 1% formaldehyde in distilled water and follow with foot powder or amolin powder.

## HAMMER TOE

*Recognition*—Toes are forced up in a claw-like position (Figure 7).

*Prevention*—Wear shoes that are of the proper length (long enough).

*Treatment*—Massage and force the joint down (Figure 7) or use felt pad (Figure 8).

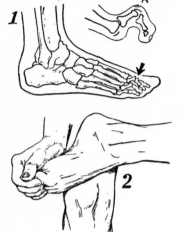

FIGURE 7. Hammer toes, showing affected skeletal structure.

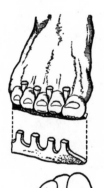

FIGURE 8a. Toe pad is cut from ¼″ felt and used to hold or support the four lesser toes. Works well on a high arched foot, or a foot with prominent metatarsal area; or for hammer toes. Reduces friction on the ends of toes. Cut thinner under big toe to help hold pad in position.

BUNION

*Recognition*—Deformed big toe joint.

*Prevention*—Wear shoes of the proper length and width.

*Treatment*—Apply pad (Figure 9), with adhesive tape. Do not tape too tightly as return to normal position must be gradual. Heat, whirlpool and Cramergesic Pack will remove soreness.

FIGURE 8b. This is similar to preceding pad. In addition to the same results as preceding pad, the ring can be shaped for either second, third, or fourth toes *to act as a padding for a painful corn.* The hole must be cut large enough for the toe to fit through without tearing the felt.

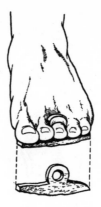

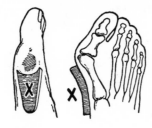

FIGURE 9. Application of Pad to Bunion.

## TRANSVERSE ARCH (METATARSAL) INJURIES

*Recognition*—Severe pain just to the inside of the ball of the foot when the individual goes up on his toes (Figure 10).

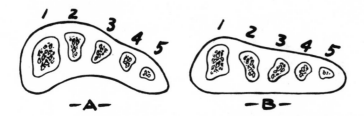

FIGURE 10a. A cross-section of the metatarsal bones of a normal transverse arch. Normal pressure is on the first and fifth bones.

FIGURE 10b. A fallen transverse arch—pressure now on the second, third, and fourth metatarsal heads.

*Prevention*—Wear proper footwear and run on a soft surface.

*Treatment*—(Figure 11).

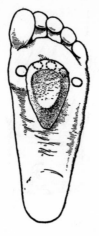

FIGURE 11a. This is the common metatarsal head pad. The important point is in the placing of the pad. The thickest part is back of the head and the feathered edge goes forward over the heads. The point of importance here is that the highest elevation is just behind the heads in order to pick them up. Use ¼″ wool or cotton felt.

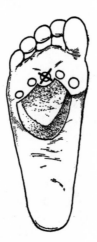

FIGURE 11b. This is a ¼″ thick felt metatarsal pad with a cut-out for a definite painful area [x]. The cut-out can be made to fit over any of the metatarsal heads desired. This takes the pressure off the painful spot and spreads it over pain-free areas.

### STRESS FRACTURE—METATARSAL

*Recognition*—Symptoms of a fallen transverse arch plus extreme tenderness and a slight swelling on top of the foot, usually the third metatarsal.

*Treatment*—Place the foot in an orthopedic shoe (Figure 6), or a plaster cast. Remove daily for 20 minutes of whirlpool treatment.

*Taping*—When doctor will permit, use an "X" strapping (Figure 12) and continue to encircle the foot snugly with adhesive

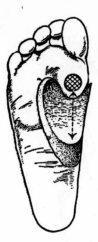

FIGURE 11c. This ¼" felt pad is used to divert pressure from a prominent big toe joint [1st metatarsal phalangeal joint], or a blistered or calloused area at this spot. Note that the pad must run down the shaft of the first metatarsal bone in order to give it support. Dotted line indicates approximate position of first metatarsal shaft.

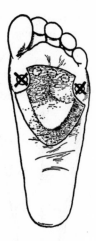

FIGURE 11d. This is a cut-out pad for the commonly seen painful area under the 1st and 5th joints. Note the pad is NOT skived [beveled] on the forward end. This is to give support through this region and keep the weight off the 1st and 5th areas.

*Every pad used should aim toward correction of improper position of the foot and must insure comfort and permit relaxation. Testing and retesting for shape and thickness will pay dividends.

tape down to base of the toes. Finish with a complete ankle strapping (Figure 18).

LONGITUDINAL ARCH

*Recognition*—Pain in the main arch of the foot.
*Taping*—Figure 12 or 13.

## "X" STRAPPING

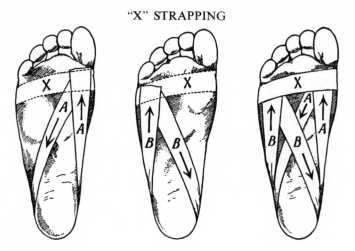

FIGURE 12. Use 1″ adhesive tape. Anchors (x) and strips (A and B) should not be snug.

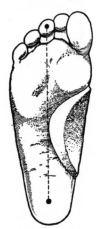

FIGURE 13. The line is drawn from the center of the third toe down to the center of the heel. This is the guiding line for placing the lateral edge of the pad. If the pad does not cross this line, the patient will not complain of discomfort. The line is merely a guide. This cue is directed for the proper placing of a pad for the longitudinal arch only.

*Foot Rest* (Addition to "X" strapping)—1 in. strip of adhesive tape around side of foot from little toe to big toe. Fill in bottom (no tension) up to side strips from base of toes to heel.

### CALLOUS

*Cause*—Incorrectly fitting shoes, friction, pressure, weakening of transverse arch, etc.

*Treatment*—Remove the cause; file the callous down with a wood rasp, sandpaper, callous file, pedicor (do not use a razor blade because of the danger of cutting into live tissue). If the callous remains sore, soak in Boric Acid or Sodium Bicarbonate Solution. To often, place a Salicylic Acid Plaster on the callous or put adhesive tape over it and leave for two to three days.

## CORN (HARD)

*Recognition*—An overgrowth of skin (callous) which dips down and presses on nerves.

*Treatment*—Remove the pressure which caused the corn. File the corn as you would file a callous. To remove the remainder of the corn, use Salicylic Acid Plaster Corn Pad. Paint with 10% salicylic acid in collodion or ordinary tape left on corn for two to three days may cause it to soften and disappear. Pad for painful corn (Figure 8).

## CORN (SOFT)

*Recognition*—A soft, white, flaky area usually with a small hole in the center. Found between the toes, usually the last two toes.

*Cause*—Excessive sweating of feet; not cleaning and drying toes thoroughly; shoes that do not fit.

*Treatment*—Eliminate the cause; wash with alcohol; paint with 5% solution of silver nitrate; powder; keep toes apart and dry with felt or cotton.

## PLANTAR'S WART

*Recognition*—A very painful area on the sole of the foot (possibly on palm of hand) at level of head of metatarsals (Figure 14B). It looks like a small oval callous with a core. To aid in diagnosis, moisten wart with alcohol. If it is a plantar's wart, there will usually be black spots under the callous.

*Cause*—Friction or the newer belief that it may be caused by a virus infection and may be mildly contagious.

*Treatment*—Usually will have to be seen by a physician. Treatments that we have used are (1) Salicylic Acid tape for three or four days, rest three to four days and repeat. (2) Soak foot in

hot water; cut a hole in a piece of moleskin; fill with 60% Salicylic Acid Ointment, Nitric Acid or Foot Ointment, remove in
three days. Coat surrounding normal skin with vaseline, etc.
(3) Metatarsal pad to relieve pain. May result in a cure. (4)
Ultra-Sound.

*Doctor's Recommendations*—Electric Needle, X-Ray.

STONE BRUISE

*Cause*—A severe bruise on bottom of heel affecting soft tissue
and possibly bone.

*Treatment*—Apply ice immediately. Second day whirlpool
and Cramergesic Packs.

*Taping*—Figure 14A and 14B.

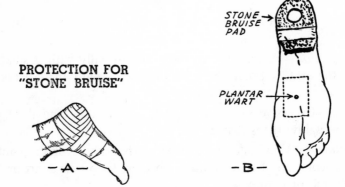

FIGURE 14a. Basketweave tape (½″ or 1″) with extreme force.
Figure 8 taping (1½″) then applied over basketweave to secure
loose ends.

FIGURE 14b. Cut a piece of sponge rubber (Figure 6) or felt (¼″)
to fit the heel—cut a hole in the rubber slightly larger than the
tender area. Secure pad to heel with adhesive tape.

*Special Protective Equipment*—Make a heel cup out of fiber
glass, castex or out of a tablespoon (cut handle off spoon; flat-
ten front and sides slightly; back part will fit contour of heel;
tape to heel; fine for protecting bruises anywhere on foot or
ankle (Figure 6). Heel cups may also be purchased from the

Wolverine Supply Company, or the MF Athletic Company (Figure 6).

*Doctor's Recommendation*—Steroid, Enzyme, Local Anesthetic.

## BLOOD BLISTER—EDGE OF HEEL

*Recognition*—A hard, crusted, dark calloused area along the edge of the heel.

*Cause*—Lateral sliding of foot in the shoe: friction, pinching.

*Treatment*—File the area as explained under treatment of callouses, whirlpool, Cramergesic Packs.

*Taping*—Same as for Stone Bruise (Figure 14A and 14B).

## HEEL SPUR—CALLOUS

*Recognition*—Pain, tenderness, swelling, callous-like enlargement on heel, just below where top of low-cut shoes stop.

*Cause*—Improper shoes; pressure; bruise; friction; injury to calcaneus (heel) bone.

*Treatment*—Whirlpool, Cramergesic Packs; Ultra-Sound.

*Taping Methods*—Cut a piece of felt in the shape of a doughnut and tape over the area. This will relieve pressure and possibly the tenderness will disappear. (2) Place a heel pad in the shoe. (3) Use tablespoon as explained under Stone Bruise.

*Doctor's Recommendations*—Surgery.

## TENOSYNOVITIS

*Recognition*—An irritation and inflammation of any tendon sheath (top of foot, achilles tendon, wrist, etc.). Feel and sometimes hear crinkly wax paper-like feeling as tendon moves in swollen sheath. Pain. Crepitation.

*Cause*—Bruise, blow, pressure, not in shape, changing from one sport to another.

*Treatment*—Heat and rest. Alternate whirlpool (108-110 degrees) and Microtherm daily. Cramergesic Packs in-between. May put in splint for complete rest, remove for heat.

*Taping*—A snug bandage with a sponge rubber heel pad.

*Doctor's Recommendations*—Skeletal Muscle Relaxant, Steroid, Enzyme, Local Anesthetic.

### ACHILLES TENDON STRAIN

*Recognition*—Pain along the tendon when toe is flexed. Occasionally where toe is extended.

*Cause*—Sudden strain or blow.

*Treatment*—Ice immediately followed by treatment rules.

*Taping*—Tape to shorten the tendon. Extend the toe and tape as illustrated in Figure 15. First strip of tape (1½ in.) starts behind ball of foot and extends up to calf. Second and third strips start on top of instep, down under heel and crosses on Achilles tendon, leaving ankle bone free. Repeat strips 1-2-3 and anchor below calf, above ankle bones and over arch. Use a sponge rubber heel pad in practice and street shoe.

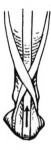

FIGURE 15. Taping to shorten the tendon. View is of the heel of the foot.

If injury pains when the toe is extended, just reverse the above taping method. Flex the toe; start first strip behind toes on top of foot and extend up the shin; second and third strips in front of the leg.

*Doctor's Recommendations*—Same as tenosynovitis.

### ANKLE SPRAIN

In a recent lecture, Dr. Don O'Donoghue of Oklahoma City made the following statements in regard to ankle injuries: "Eighty-five per cent of ankle injuries are inversion injuries." (Figure 16B). He further went on to classify their diagnosis

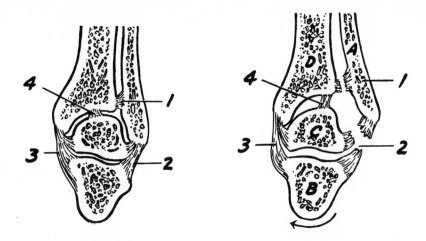

FIGURE 16a. View of a normal right ankle (from rear) showing ligaments that may be sprained. (1) Anterior Tibiofibular Ligament. (2) Lateral Collateral Ligament. (Calcaneofibular). (3) Medical Collateral (Deltoid) Ligament. (4) Anterior Astragalus—Tibial Ligament.

FIGURE 16b. Diagrammatic figure of most commonly sprained ligaments. (A) Fibula. (B) Calcaneum. (C) Astrangalus or Talus. (D) Tibia.

---

and treatment as follows:

A. Type of Injury

    1. Inversion (inversion, internal rotation, plantar flexion).

    2. Eversion (eversion, external rotation, dorsal flexion).

B. Diagnosis

    History—Time of injury; manner of injury; direction of force; degree of disability, time of onset; pain, swelling; whether or not deformity was corrected.

C. Examination

    1. Observation—Deformity, discoloration, swelling.

    2. Palpitation—Tension of skin, crepitation, range of motion, abnormal motion.

    3. X-ray.

D. Degree of Injury

1. Mild—Partial ligament tear, no loss of strength.

2. Moderate—Complete tear of part of ligament with loss of strength.

3. Severe complete tear of ligament with complete loss of strength.

E. Mild Sprain

1. Diagnosis—Local swelling, tenderness, pain and mild disability, X-ray negative.

2. Treatment—Pressure, ice, local injection, heat, strapping, and continued activity.

F. Moderate Sprain

1. Diagnosis—More pain, swelling, disability, and pain on reproducing stress and on normal motion, X-ray negative.

2. Treatment—Designed to prevent further injury: pressure and ice (30 minutes to overnight), injection, heat (no sooner than ten hours), splints, walking cast, strapping.

G. Severe Sprain

1. Diagnosis—Positive: severe early swelling, pain and disability. Pain on normal motion. Abnormal motion possible. Possible X-ray findings.

2. Treatment—

a. Non-surgical: same as moderate sprain.

b. Surgical: complete repair, splint ten days, walking cast ten days, strap.

*Prevention*—An ounce of prevention is worth a pound of cure. For this reason we require all of our boys (football and basketball) to wear the Louisiana Lock Ankle Wrap (Figure 17). We feel that by wearing this ankle wrap, if a boy's ankle is injured, it will be one degree less than it would have been had he not had the wrap on. Other schools have had fine success by requiring their boys to wear ankle wraps. In a survey made at Harvard University and reported in the American Medical Association

Journal of December 14, 1946, Drs. T. B. Quigley, James Cox and Joseph Murphy stated that since they had started the routine use of ankle wraps (15 years) none of their athletes had suffered a complete ankle ligament rupture. Dr. D. F. Hanley of Bowdoin College phrased it a little differently when he said, "We have not lost a man for a game in five years who has worn his ankle wraps correctly." Ankle wraps are 2¼ in. wide and 96 in. in length. They can be purchased in 72-yard rolls and cut to desired lengths (Figure 6).

TAPING

We prefer to use a basketweave with a heel-lift using 1½ in. tape. All of our taping is done directly to the skin (taping rules, Chapter VI).

If we are taping for preventive purposes, we have the boy hold his foot so it is perpendicular to the floor. If we are trying to protect a lateral sprain, we instruct the athlete to hold his foot perpendicular with a slight outward rotation (shorten ligaments on lateral side of ankle). Reverse procedure if injury is to inside of ankle. The following views refer to the illustration in Figure 18 (pg. 80).

VIEW 1. Start the first perpendicular strip of tape a minimum of 4" above the ankle bone on the inside rear of the leg, carry it down under the heel and up the outside of the leg to just below the calf (VIEW 2). The first circular strip starts just above the ankle bone and completely encircles the leg.

VIEW 2. Second perpendicular strip overlaps the first, from a fanning top to more of an overlap over the joint. Second circular strip overlaps circular strip number one.

VIEW 3. Third perpendicular and circular strips follow same lines (overlapping) as the second strips.

VIEW 4. Fourth circular strip anchors top of perpendicular strips.

VIEW 5. Circular strips 5-6-7 overlap each other as they work down the leg from circular strip number 4. Start of heel-lift.

VIEW 6. Complete ankle-taping. Be especially sure you do not leave any open spaces along the Achilles tendon or it will cause a pinching or blistering.

For prevention, it is possible to use tape instead of an ankle wrap when applying a Louisiana Heel Lock (Figure 17).

## LOUISIANA ANKLE WRAP*

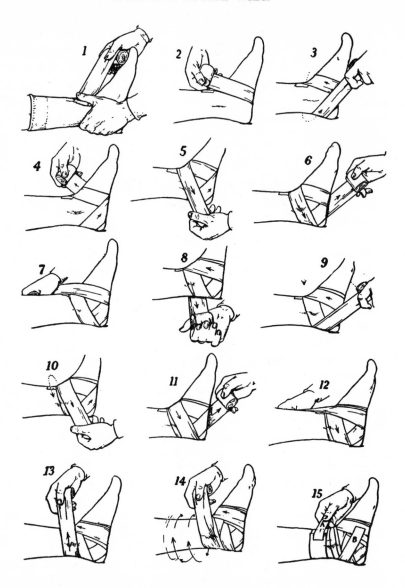

FIGURE 17. "Louisiana Ankle Wrap." Apply over a sweat sock. The sock will act as a cushion against cutting into the skin.

The wrap is approximately 96 inches long. No. 1 starts on top, but here again there is a difference of opinion. Some start around the foot, some around the leg. We don't consider this difference of opinion vital, as the wrap will equalize itself.

Follow the diagram as illustrated from figures No. 1 to and including No. 15.

In No. 13, the "heel-lock" is completed and the balance of the wrap is carried around the leg (No. 14) to afford a cushion against bruising blows.

In No. 15, the end of the wrap is secured snugly with a 3-inch strip of tape—illustrated "A." "B" is a strip of tape 10 or 11 inches long. It starts toward the front, is carried over the triangle formed by the 3 directions of wrap, back in the heel depression and on the outside, over the other triangle and to the front.

The application of the "B" tape anchor is extremely important because it stabilizes the entire wrap, especially over the Achilles Tendon area where additional protection is needed.

After you learn the principle of the wrap, the rest is easy. You will soon learn to apply the correct amount of tension.

We suggest that you learn it yourself, then teach it to your players. Then have them pair off and wrap each other's ankles. In this way you will cut the length to approximately 84."

One loop around each side of the heel instead of the two illustrated will cut the length to approximately 84."

---

*Courtesy Cramer Chemical Co.

SPECIAL PROTECTIVE EQUIPMENT

For an extremely weak ankle, we will incorporate a felt horse shoe, as illustrated in Figure 6, on the injured side of the ankle. This will permit freedom of flexion and extension, but will prevent inversion or eversion.

To determine if an ankle is strong enough to practice, run in circles to right and left. If there is no limp, the boy should be able to practice.

*Doctor's Recommendations*—Enzyme, Steroids.

*Rehabilitative Exercises*—See Chapter XV for specific exercises for ankle, arch and lower leg.

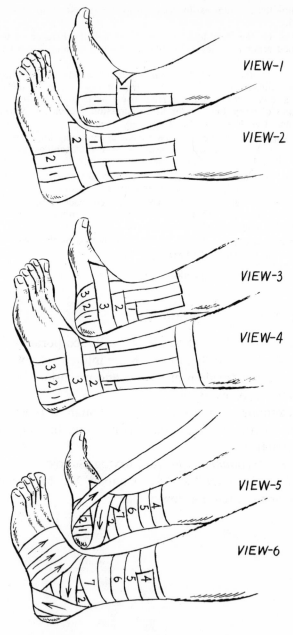

FIGURE 18. Taping procedure. See page 77 for description of views.

# CHAPTER X

# Lower Leg, Knee, and Thigh Conditions and Injuries

## SHIN SPLINTS

*Recognition*—Pain on either side of lower 1/3 of shin bone. Often can feel a roughened area (similar to small grains of sand) along the bone as one gently runs his finger up and down the bone.

*Cause*—In dealing with shin splints, one is dealing with a multitude of different causes. All of the causes could be true. Some of the beliefs are that shin splints are due to a dropping of the arch which sets up a reaction in the five tendons of the lower leg; irritation of interosseus membrane (between tibia and fibula); an inflammation (many minute ruptures of muscle) of the tibial periosteum; muscle spasm caused by swelling of anterior tibial muscle; a strain of soleus or tibialis posterior muscle; periostitis at attachment of tibialis muscle to tibial crest. Other causes are lised under prevention.

*Prevention*—(1) Start early (arches strapped) and work gradually into shape. (2) Run low on the foot, do not get up on the toes. (3) Run in tennis shoes (no spikes). (4) Beware of hard surfaces, run on grass. (5) Reverse directions as you run—not always to your left. (6) Run backwards. (7) Rock from heel to toe. (8) On back, raise right leg perpendicularly and touch opposite left hip with head and shoulders flat. Repeat with left

81

leg. (9) On back, grasp knees and pull up to chin. Rock back and forth. (10) Sitting, extend foot with toes curled and grasp trainer's hand. Trainer forces foot back against resistance. Repeat, starting with foot flexed.

*Treatment*—There is nothing better than complete rest and heat around the clock (whirlpool 106-108 degrees, hydrocollator, lamps, Cramergesic Packs on shin and low back). You cannot run out shin splints. Wear a sponge heel pad at all times. We have a ruling that we will not tape a boy's shin unless he can get twenty minutes of heat before practicing.

*Taping*—There are almost as many methods as there are trainers. In our preferred method, we start by applying an "x" longitudinal arch strapping (Figure 12). We continue with the method illustrated in Figure 19, and we will finish with a figure eight ankle wrap put on in reverse so as to lift the arch (this is optional).

Other methods of support are:

1. Apply a double weave, same as Figure 19, only alternate the starting point from the outside to the inside, etc.

2. Place a piece of sponge rubber 1 in. wide along the shin and hold snugly with adhesive tape or an elastic wrap (Figure 6).

3. Tape a felt pad under arch and big toe (Figure 6).

4. Extend the ankle and apply three 1½ in. strips of tape around the ball of the foot, then flex the ankle tightly and apply two strips around the shin 3 in. above the ankle bone.

5. Elastic stocking.

6. Start 1½ in. tape at base of fifth metatarsal (prominent bone on outside of foot). Bring under foot and up inside of leg and cross over and finish under head of fibula (outside of leg). Repeat on other side if necessary. Finish with rest strapping.

*Doctor's Recommendation*—Enzyme, Vitamin B₁₂.

### Varicose Vein

A problem for the team physician. However, a boy can be given relief if he will wear an elastic stocking.

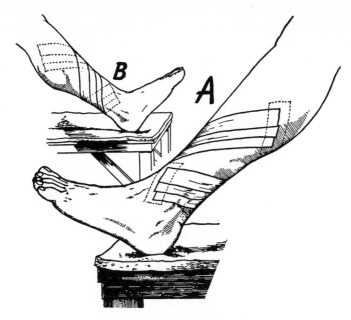

FIGURE 19. *Shin Splint.* Start on the outside of the leg just above the ankle with 1½" adhesive tape. Spiral behind the leg, and as you come to the shin area use your free hand to push the excess skin and tissue in towards the shin bone. Then as tape comes across the irritated shin it will hold the above tissue, protecting it from further irritation. Anchor tape at top and bottom as indicated by dotted lines. Figure B indicates how it will look from the opposite side. If desired, entire area can then be wrapped with an elastic wrap. If irritation is on the outside of the shin, reverse the above procedure. If both sides of the shin are injured, apply a double weave—same as above, only alternate the starting point from outside to inside, etc.

## MUSCLE CRAMPS—HEAT CRAMPS

*Recognition*—A severe contraction of any muscle in the body.

*Causes*—Fatigue; lack of salt, vitamin C or calcium; sudden exposure to cold; muscle made to do things to which it is un-accustomed; improper warm up; lack of stretching exercises.

*Prevention*—Graduated stretching exercises throughout the pre-season and season. Salt tablets and Vitamin C. We have available in our training room after each early season practice a cool saline solution (8-10 tablespoons salt to 10 gal. water).

We feel this has helped in the prevention of muscular cramps, and heat exhaustion. We also feel that our boys eat a better meal after practice if they drink a cup of saline solution. It seems to quench their thirst so they can eat rather than just sit at the table and drink iced tea or lemonade.

*Treatment*—Relieving muscle cramps (1) Lengthen the muscle. Stretch it. (2) Restore the circulation. Heat and vigorous massage. (3) Salt, calcium, and vitamin C.

*Doctor's Recommendation*—Skeletal Muscle Relaxants.

Why take salt tablets? The drinking of large quantities of water without a proportionate intake of salt is harmful in that it leads to more profuse sweating and a greater loss of salt from the body. Salt ingestion is essential for proper tissue metabolism for the body tissues cannot store salt. It must be replaced daily.

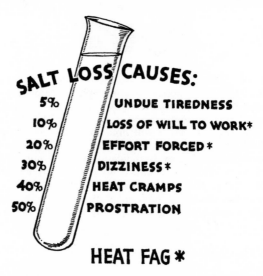

**SALT LOSS CAUSES:**

| | |
|---|---|
| 5% | **UNDUE TIREDNESS** |
| 10% | **LOSS OF WILL TO WORK*** |
| 20% | **EFFORT FORCED*** |
| 30% | **DIZZINESS*** |
| 40% | **HEAT CRAMPS** |
| 50% | **PROSTRATION** |

**HEAT FAG ***

FIGURE 20. "The Why of Salt." Daily sweating, during practice, carries away excessive amounts of salt. This loss of salt disturbs the delicate metabolic processes that are responsible for converting food elements into energy for exercise. *Body tissue cannot store salt. It must be replaced, daily!*

*EVERY ATHLETE WHO SWEATS NEEDS SALT.* Excessive sweating flushes the salt out of your tissues. The more water you drink, without taking salt, the more you sweat and the more salt you flush out. *This process becomes a vicious circle, repeating itself . . . day after day.*

SALT LOSS CAUSES: 5% undue tiredness, 10% loss of will to work*, 20% effort forced*, |30% |dizziness*, 40% |heat cramps, 50% prostration.
  *Heat fag.

*Courtesy Cramer Chemical Co.

## OSGOOD-SCHLATTER KNEE FRACTURE

*Recognition*—It is actually not a fracture and it is not a knee injury. It is a forcible separation of the tibial tubercle. (Tibial tubercle is the projection of the anterior head of the tibia. In youth, the connection between the main bone and the head of the bone is soft. It hardens with age). When the athlete sits on a table and bends his knee, the bone pushes out into the flesh (Figure 21). It goes back in place when the leg is straight.

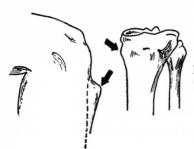

FIGURE 21. Osgood-Schlatter knee fracture. -

*Cause*—An injury of early teen-aged youths, due to a blow, jumping, or disease.

*Treatment*—Relieve the pain and tenderness. Whirlpool, microtherm, hydrocollator, ultra-sound with Cramergesic packs in between.

*Taping*—With the athlete standing, tape snugly immediately below the tibial projection (may use a felt pressure pad below injury). Finish by completely encircling that area of the leg with elastic adhesive tape.

*Protective Equipment*—Athlete should always wear at least a sponge rubber knee pad. It may be necessary to improvise a doughnut pad out of plastic or make a pad out of castex or fiber glass so as to keep the pressure off the injured area.

*Doctor's Recommendation*—If the injury is discovered early enough a splint can be placed on the back of the leg. This will prevent the knee from bending long enough to permit the fracture to heal (3-5 weeks). Another possibility is surgery.

KNEE INJURIES

In Figure 22 the two main bones of the knee (femur and tibia) have been separated to show the articular surfaces between the bones with the semilunar cartilages C and D. A. and B. are the anterior and posterior cruciate ligaments. They are called cruciate because they cross each other like the lines of a letter X. E. is the patellar ligament with the infra-patellar bursae (a sack containing fluid found or formed over an exposed and prominent part, or where a tendon plays over a bone—approximately 13 in and around the joint). The cruciates are two of the ten ligaments which hold the joint in position.

Figure 23 shows what may happen when an athlete is clipped from the outside of the knee as shown by the single arrow. The

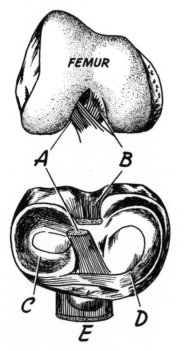

FIGURE 22. View of normal knee.

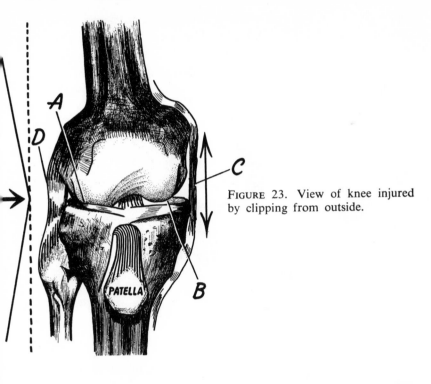

FIGURE 23. View of knee injured by clipping from outside.

dotted line indicates normal relationship while the solid line illustrates the angle produced by the blow. The figure shows the increase of pressure on the lateral cartilage at A and the release of pressure at B—with the double arrow showing over-extension of the medial collateral ligament. The patella (knee cap) has been turned down on its ligament revealing the articular surface of the knee cap and the femur. The medial collateral ligament C is long and fan-shaped, is part of the joint capsule and its deep layer is attached to the medial cartilage. The lateral collateral ligament D is long and cord-like; it is not a part of the capsule and the lateral cartilage is not attached to it.

A knee demands *early*, careful examination. Dr. Don O'Donoghue believes you should note especially:

(1) Severity of injury, (2) degree of disability, (3) abnormal motion, (4) location of tenderness, (5) amount and rapidity of swelling, (6) restriction of pain on normal motion, (7) locking.

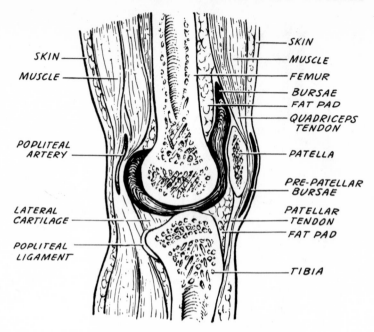

FIGURE 24. Knee Joint—Longitudinal Cross section, Lateral View.

He further states that the severity of the knee injury may be mild, moderate or severe.  For example:

A. Mild—some fibers of ligament damaged, no loss of strength of ligament.

B. Moderate—Definite tear in ligament, loss of strength.

C. Severe—Complete tear of ligaments and complete loss of integrity.

The symptoms for a mild knee sprain are classified into two groups, positive and negative.

A. Positive—(1) tender at site of tear, (2) pain on abnormal stress, (3) local swelling, (4) pain on forced motion.

B. Negative—(1) no instability, (2) no blood in joint, (3) no effusion, (4) no locking, (5) no pain on normal motion.

Treatment for the mild knee sprain is: (1) rest, (2) cold, then heat, (3) protection, (4) injection (local, enzyme, steroid, procaine, etc.), (5) early active motion, (6) no immobilization.

The common symptoms for the moderate knee sprain are:

. A. Positive—(1) pain in knee, (2) local tenderness, (3) disability, (4) swelling, (5) fluid in joint, (6) pain on stress, (7) locking.

B. Negative—no abnormal mobility.

The treatment for the moderate knee sprain is: (1) pressure, (2) cold, then heat, (3) rest, (4) aspiration of joint, (5) injection of joint, (6) protection (splint, cast, tape), (7) rehabilitation (very important).

The symptoms for a severe knee sprain are: (1) immediate disability, (2) knee gives away, (3) severe pain, (4) abnormal motion, (5) blood in joint, (6) blood infiltration, (7) marked swelling, (8) locking, (9) positive X-ray.

The non-surgical treatment for the severe knee sprain is the same as the moderate sprain. The surgical treatment for the severe knee sprain is: (1) prompt decision, (2) early repair, (3) complete repair of all ligaments torn, (4) repair, not reconstruction.

## KNEE INJURIES

*Prevention*—We prefer that all our boys wear oblong cleats in practice (Figure 32) as we feel this will help to cut down on injuries to the knee.

*Examination*—Be systematic, and thorough; watch the eyes, they will indicate pain; check the patella; compare the knees (contour, discoloration, swelling—hot indicates infection); check joint-line (cartilage groove) and ligaments from origin to insertion (if torn, there will be a roughness like particles of sand or rice); check size of quadriceps for atrophy (indication of an old injury).

All knee tests must be modified to fit the conditions, including swelling, tenderness, and stiffness. The test should be carried out with the knee straight and also with a slight bend in the knee with the muscles relaxed and with the muscles flexed. The important test is the test with the knee straight. Start all tests on the good knee. This will give the patient confidence that you are not going to hurt him and you can also use it for comparison. The cartilage and joint-line are one and the same thing.  While checking a knee, keep one hand on or as close as possible to this joint line all the time.  You may pick up a crackling, clicking sensation which will indicate a cartilage injury or a joint mouse and you will also be able to feel joint movement.

*Ligament Tests*—Figure 25-26-27-28.

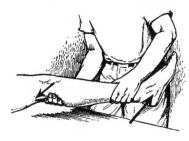

FIGURE 25.  Medial collateral ligament test.  Grasp leg with both hands as pictured.  Attempt to move lower leg toward you, holding knee steady.  Do not use force.  Look for excessive tenderness and joint movement.

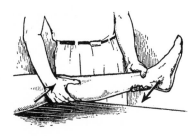

FIGURE 26.  Lateral collateral ligament test.  As pictured, attempt to move the lower leg away from you, holding the knee steady.

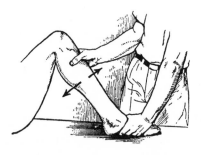

FIGURE 27.  Cruciate ligament test.  Check forward and backward motion in the joint (drawer test).  This test may also be accomplished by letting the knee drop over the end of the table (as in figure 29) and then checking the forward and backward motion.  There is normally a ¼″ movement.

*Cartilage Tests*—(1) Any of the ligament tests, (2) Figure 29. (3) Diagnosis of torn medial cartilage is often clinched by the following maneuver: Patient in sitting position, ask him to put a little weight on the heel of the involved side, then slowly rotate

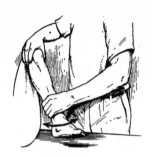

FIGURE 28. An over all test—ligaments and cartilage. Use different degrees of pressure with right hand while moving lower leg with left hand. Check for grating and looseness.

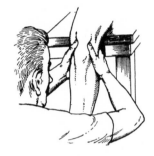

FIGURE 29. Cartilage test. Place thumb against lower edge of the patella and move gently along the joint line as you lightly rotate, flex and extend the leg.

his foot outward. Pain along the medial joint line makes one suspicious of a torn medial cartilage. When the foot is rotated inward, pain on lateral joint indicates a possible injured lateral cartilage. (4) Locking: (a) torn cartilage, (b) joint mouse—a small section of bone, cartilage or ex-soft tissue broken off from its attachment. This mouse floats all around the knee and may cause an irritation or locking of the joint. Torn cartilage (Figure 32).

*Reduction of Displaced Cartilage*—Medial cartilage is injured six to eight times more frequently than the lateral cartilage. Often it is possible to slip a cartilage back into its groove. However, there are occasions when a knee becomes locked and it is impossible to unlock it manually. If this should occur, the knee will require surgery.

1. Patient sitting on table, leg over side of table, relax and swing the leg forward and backward and at the same time add internal and external rotation, alternately. This enlarges the joint and tends to loosen the cartilage.

2. Slowly flex and extend the knee with light outward and inward pressure.

3. The trainer places his arm behind the knee joint and slowly flexes the knee (this will open up the joint) and then exert light outward and inward pressure.

4. Patient on his back. Trainer grasps patient's ankle and exerts a light pull (traction) on the leg while lightly rotating the knee in and out.

5. Patient on his back. Trainer flexes knee to chest. If a medial cartilage, place one hand on the arch of the foot and gently pull the leg out laterally, and at the same time exert inward pressure with the other hand (fingers on cartilage line if possible). Shake the knee. With leg in this position (external rotation) bring it out into full extension.

6. Same as Number 5. Only rotate the knee in outward and inward circles while flexed on the chest (fingers on joint-line as this may enable you to push the cartilage back in). Finish by bringing knee to extension as in Number 5.

TAPING METHOD

We use a double weave (inside and outside of joint) with 3 in. elastic adhesive tape. If additional support is necessary, we will:

1. Incorporate regular adhesive with the elastic tape.
2. Include a felt pressure pad (Figure 32) on the weak side of the knee put on after strip #8.
3. Incorporate the taping for an over-extended knee (Figure 31) along with the regular knee-taping method.

We determine the amount of flexion and extension we will permit by the angle of the knee joint at the start of the taping (straighter the knee, the less movement), and by the tension we place on the elastic tape (for a tight taping, take all the elastic stretch out of the tape). The tape should come quite close to the patella, but should not touch it at any time. If you are taping with regular and adhesive tape, fold the edges over as they cross the knee joint to prevent the tape from tearing.

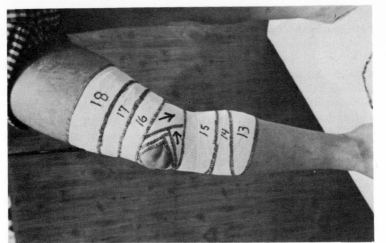

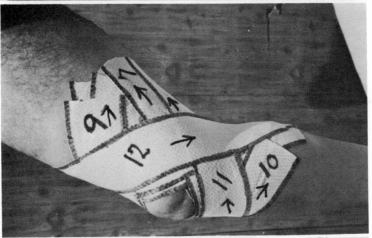

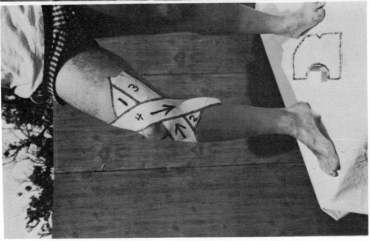

FIGURE 30. Taping knee injury.

VIEW 1. Strip #1 starts on the lateral side of the leg, behind the calf and angles up above the patella (as close as possible to the patella) and ends on the inside of the thigh. Strip #2 starts on the outside of the thigh, angles below the patella (as close as possible) and ends behind the calf on or near the start of strip #1. Strip #3 starts behind the calf on the outside of the leg and angles up under the patella (as close as possible) and ends on the inside of the thigh. Strip #4 starts on the outside of the thigh, angles down above the patella (as close as possible) and the ends behind the calf of leg.

VIEW 2. Basketweave strips 4-5-6-7-8-9-10-11-12 over and same angles as strips 1-2-3-4 with a considerable overlap of each strip. Strips 1-5-9 follow the same contour and angle as do strips 2-6-10; 3-7-11 and 4-8-12.

VIEW 3. Encircle the leg starting at calf with strips 13-14-15. Leave popiteal area open (space behind knee joint) and encircle leg above knee joint with strips 16-17-18.

*Doctor's Recommendation*—Most doctors prefer to remove a torn cartilage (Figure 32) as it is composed of fibro-cartilage which does not repair itself, and therefore recurrence is certain and eventual removal will be necessary. Aspirate (drain) any fluid that may be present. Drugs used for various types of knee injuries: Steroids, Enzymes.

HYPEREXTENSION TEST

Knee straight. Support ankles with left hand and with very gentle force, press down on knee cap. Pain in back of knee will indicate over-extension.

CRUCIATE LIGAMENTS OR HYPEREXTENSION (Figure 27)
    TAPING METHOD (Figure 31 A and B)

FLUID ON KNEE

A good way of detecting this is by the "Patellar Click." With the knee straight, place one hand palm down over the lower end of the quadriceps (approximately one inch above the patella) with light pressure toward the toes. With index finger of other hand, gently press the patella down, release it and press down again. If fluid (water) is present, one will experience a click similar to two ice cubes striking together in a glass of water.

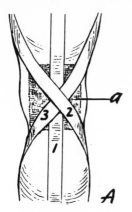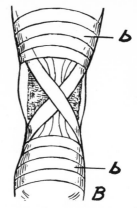

FIGURE 31a, b. Player standing with a 2″ pad under heel to keep his knee slightly flexed. "a"—felt or gauze pad on back of knee to prevent cutting in popliteal area. 1-2-3 are the first three strips of 1½″ or 2″ regular adhesive tape—continue to basketweave the tape; overlapping the first three strips. Follow with circular strips of three-inch elastic (b) adhesive tape around the leg.

The above wrap can also be used under or over the collateral or cartilage taping (Figure 30) to add strength and support.

*Treatment*—In treatment of fluid on the knee, follow the rules in Chapter VII with special emphasis on pressure and ice. Follow above treatment with a pressure bandage over sponge rubber compress (Figure 32).

*Doctor's Recommendation*—Aspirate (removal of fluid). This should be done as soon as possible, one way or another. Steroids, Enzymes.

KNEE BRACES

We personally prefer to tape our knees, however, we do at times use the following mechanical braces:
Octopus; Clam (especially in wrestling); Peckham; Olympic Champion (Figure 32).

TESTS TO DETERMINE IF KNEE IS STRONG ENOUGH TO PRACTICE:

1. The motor for the knee is the quadriceps (thigh) muscle. It runs the knee joint. If it is well developed, the knee will go. If not, it will collapse. The circumference of the thigh above the injured knee should be equal to or greater than the circumference of the opposite thigh. This can be determined by: (a) measuring eight inches up the thigh from the top of the knee cap and then measuring the circumference (some feel this is not an accu-

95

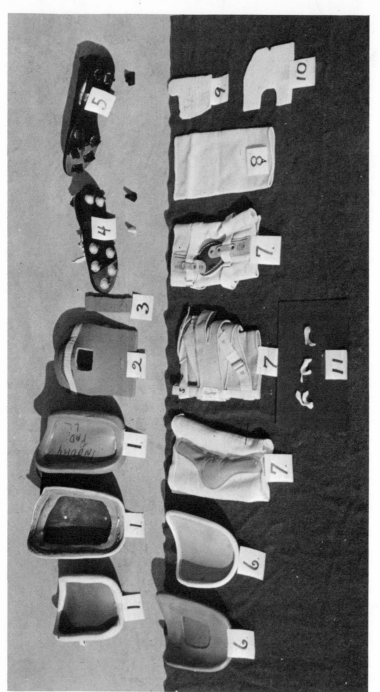

FIGURE 32. Protective equipment (Lower Leg—Knee—Thigh).

1. Thigh injury pads
2. Sponge rubber knee compress
3. Sponge shin splint strip
4. Game shoe with game cleats
5. Practice shoe with oblong cleats
6. Thigh pads
7. Knee braces
8. Thigh Cap
9. Shin splint pad—under arch and big toe
10. Felt knee pressure pad
11. Torn knee cartilages

rate way of testing as it is possible to elevate the patella from ½ to ¾ of an inch); (b) measure from the anterior-superior end of the spine of the pelvis 10 to 15 inches down the thigh and then measure the circumference.

2. Running tests as described under ankles (Chapter IX).

3. There are different theories on weight lifting: (a) lift 85 lbs. once or (b) lift 55 lbs. twice or (c) lift 50 lbs. 10 times in 40 seconds.

*Rehabilitative Exercises*—See Chapter XV.

### CHARLEY HORSE

A Charley horse or muscle contusion is a bruise type of injury. It is caused by a blow from the outside which damages the soft tissues, blood vessels, nerves, and may cause the muscle to go into spasm. It differs completely from a strain or pull.

*Recognition*—Tenderness, inability to run fast, possibility of a lump or muscular spasm. It is possible in a deep Charley horse to damage the periosteum of the bone. If so, in the process of repair there may be a calcification in the muscle or on the bone. This condition is called myositis ossificans and usually does not show on an X-ray for three to four weeks. This is a problem for the team physician (See Chapter XIV) (Upper Arm Bruise).

*Prevention*—Wear thigh pads slightly to the outside of the legs.

*Treatment*—If possible, have the player immediately kneel down and stretch the muscle (catcher's position) or fold leg under his body and sit on it. This prevents muscle contraction and hemorrhage. Follow with pressure bandage, ice (with knee in full flexion), and general treatment rules. The player should start to jog as soon as possible as it will aid in recovering unless it is a *very* severe injury.

*Taping Method* (Figure 33)—Patient standing, heel elevated 1½ inches. Use 1½-inch tape and start the semi-circular strapping well below and work upward (overlapping each strip) over and above the injury. Then apply diagonal (X) strips from the lower corners to the upper corners. Finish by encircling the leg with 3-inch elastic tape or an elastic thigh cap (Figure 32).

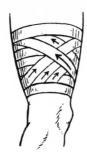

FIGURE 33. Taping Charley horse.

*Doctor's Recommendation*—Enzymes, Skeletal Muscle Relaxants, Steroids.

*Protective Equipment*—Build up the edges of the thigh pad to leave an air space between the leg and thigh pad where the injury is located (Figure 32).

*Exercises*—Under thigh in Chapter XV.

HAMSTRING STRAIN, SPRAIN

May occur in the belly or tendon of the muscle. Usually no advance warning and have a tendency to recur as fibrous scar tissue replaces the muscle tissue.

*Recognition*—Patient will give a history of a sharp, snapping sensation and will be able to point out the exact spot of the pain. Often the athlete will fall or it will be necessary for him to stop his activity immediately. About the third day the leg will discolor below site of the injury. If the injury is a mild strain, the muscle will tighten and the athlete will have to slow up.

*Causes:*

1. I feel that many so-called strains are mental. They are used as a crutch by many athletes.
2. A careless care-free warm-up (one should warm up again if more than one half-hour between events).
3. Not in condition.
4. A lack of stretching exercises.
5. Fatigue cramps. Result in loss of oxygenation.

6. Lack of salt causes muscle cramp, fatigue.
7. A sudden change in temperature causes a muscle contraction.
8. A sudden change of directions, loss of stride.

*Treatment*—General Treatment rules plus Cramergesic Pack on low back.

*Functional Tests*—(1) Athlete on his back. Trainer places one hand on the boy's knee to keep it straight and with the other hand holding the ankle he attempts to raise the leg to a right angle. Can determine the severity of the injury by the extent of height the leg can be raised. Compare with good leg. (2) Athlete squats down with arms between legs and finger tips on the floor. Raise the buttocks up so the legs are straight.

*Taping Methods*—Always wear a sponge heel pad on the leg affected. There are many trainers that do not believe in taping a hamstring strain. We, however, do use the following methods:

1. If the strain is in the belly of the muscle, we use the same taping method as explained under Charley horse (Figure 33) with the exception that we place a piece of felt 5 by 8 by ¼ in. right over the injured area before we start taping. This acts as a pressure pad. Also, we apply the encircling strips with an uplifting stress. Try to lift the belly of the muscle and shorten the pull. Finish by encircling the leg with 3-inch elastic adhesive or an elastic thigh cap (Figure 32).

2. If a light strain is in the belly of the muscle, we encircle the leg with a 2-inch strip of adhesive 2 inches above the knee and then place another strip around the leg just under the buttocks.

3. If the pull is in the tendon (under buttocks) we strap as in figure 34.

*Test to Determine if Ready to Participate*—When he can do the functional tests.

*Doctor's Recommendation*—Skeletal Muscle Relaxants, Steroids (if in tendon), Enzymes.

*Specific Exercises*—Chapter XV

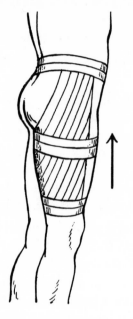

FIGURE 34. Taping tendon pull (under buttocks).

### THIGH (QUADRICEPS) STRAINS, SPRAINS

Usually in a heavy-muscled boy. Recognition, cause, treatment, and doctor's recommendations are very similar to hamstring strains.

*Functional Tests*—(1) Athlete on table on his back. Trainer, holding athlete's ankle, slowly flexes the knee and moves the heel toward the buttocks. Watch the buttocks to see if it rises or tightens for compensating purpose. (2) On back and have the athlete do quadriceps (thigh) setting exercises; if he can't, strain is probably quite severe.

*Specific Exercises*—Chapter XV.

# CHAPTER XI

# Groin, Pelvis, Buttocks, Back

### GROIN STRAIN

*Recognition*—Usually occurs in the depression between the abdomen and thigh, specifically in the Iliopsoas, Gracilis or Adductor Longus muscles. Symptoms are tenderness, cannot run fast, jump or twist.

*Cause*—Not in condition or warmed-up legs forced into a "split," poor posture.

*Treatment*—General Treatment Rules: (1) Alternate moist heat and microtherm with Cramergesic Packs on groin and low back. (2) Stretch the opposite side of the back (or both sides) as illustrated in Figure 34A. This will level the hips, and help restore normal body balance. The stretch is long-ways, no twisting motion and is not intended to be an adjustment.

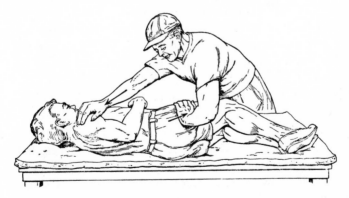

FIGURE 34a. Levelling hips to relieve groin strain.

101

(3) Often, because of improper body balance, one leg will be slightly longer than the other, usually the right. To check for this condition, place the athlete on his back with your thumbs on his ankle bones or measure from iliac crest to ankle bone (maleolus). To correct this, we use what is known as the "x" method of stretching (definitely not an adjustment or a vertebra popping) (Figure 35). Athlete on his right side; arm under head; knees drawn up (left knee flexed slightly more than right). With the athlete relaxed, rock his hip gently forward and gently push up and back on the shoulders.

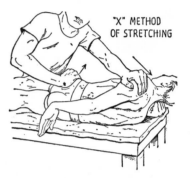

"X" METHOD
OF STRETCHING

FIGURE 35. "x" method of stretch-ing.

(4) Patient's stretch (same effect as "x" stretch). On back on table, left leg perpendicular, lay it relaxed across body (just hanging). Take a deep breath and as you exhale, relax all over. Leg will drop after each breath. Shoulders on table throughout. (5) Patient on back. Trainer will slowly stretch injured leg out laterally as far as patient will permit. Then have subject bring leg back to starting point as trainer offers resistance with body. (6) Standing beside training table, lift leg up and put foot on table (upward pressure tends to push twisted pelvis back in place). (7) Build up heel of shoe on affected side.

*Functional Test*—Rotate the foot laterally while holding the knee stiff. Lift the leg. If it is a groin strain, this will cause the patient pain.

*Taping*—Patient standing, foot elevated two inches, buttocks dropped slightly with knee and thigh rotated slightly inward so as to pull leg toward midline of the body and thus shorten all tissues in the region of the groin. Using a Charley horse wrap or two 4-inch elastic wraps or a sling-shot (made out of line rubber and used at Oklahoma—Figure 39), start the bandage high around the thigh, then figure-eight it across abdomen. The pull or lift is exerted when the bandage comes up under the buttocks across front of thigh and abdomen. Finish by pulling an elastic thigh cap up to groin. This will add support and also hold the bandage in place. It may be necessary to use the above bandage over a pair of white cotton trunks to prevent chafing.

*Doctor's Recommendation*—Skeletal Muscle Relaxant, Steroids.

*Specific Exercises*—Numbers 2, 3, 4, 5, 6 under treatment. Exercises numbers 4, 5, 6 under Hamstring Exercises and number 2, 3, 4 under Thigh Exercises. Also leg, groin, hip, back exercises in Chapter XV.

## LYMPH GLANDS

Located along the lymphatic system throughout the body. Their duty is to clear the lymph of bacteria, preventing entrance into the blood stream. In athletics, they are seen as lumps in the groin, under the arm, and under the jaw. When they occur, check the area that drains into the inflamed gland. It may be due to a local or chronic infection. Consult the physician immediately.

## BLOW TO TESTICLES

A common painful injury.

*Treatment*—(1) Lift the relaxed athlete (Figure 36) four to six inches and drop him and repeat. Object is to eliminate the muscular spasm by the sudden "jar." I have found it quite successful.

(2) Athlete on his back. Push knees up to chin keeping them 15 inches apart. (3) Loosen belt. (4) Cold towel to testicles. Never heat.

## JOCK ITCH

An irritation (dermatitis) in the region of the groin. Redness, swelling, heat and pain.

*Treatment*—(1) Make sure there is no soap on the area,

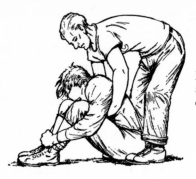

FIGURE 36. Lifting and dropping athlete to eliminate muscular spasm caused by blow to testicles.

irrigate thoroughly with water. (2) Apply Pragmatar, Desenex, Sopronol, Zinc Oxide, Mexsana Cream, or paint with Nitrotan for three days and then with Tuf Skin on the fourth day. Ultraviolet light is also effective. (3) Do not wear jockey shorts. (4) In competition, wear a soft-pouched athletic supporter, over white trunks if you wish.

### CRABS

A form of body lice that resembles a crab, and clutches the skin very closely. Usually in pubic area, under the arm and possibly on the abdomen. Bite produces intense itching. Contracted from toilet seats, benches, clothes. Treat with Cuprex.

### HEMORRHOID-PILES

Are dilated veins in the lower inch or two of the rectum. They are usually caused by constipation or strain.

*Treatment*—Keep the bowels loose and open (prunes, fruit). Wash the area at least once a day and use a soft toilet tissue. To temporarily relieve the itching, use Pazo Ointment or Nupercainal. Athlete should be sent to the team physician.

### HIP POINTER (*Bruised Crest of Ilium*)

*Recognition*—A very painful injury. A bruising or tearing of the muscle fibers and attachments along the crest of the Ilium. The bone may also be bruised or chipped. It will be painful for the athlete to cough, sneeze, laugh, twist or bend his body away from the injury.

*Cause*—A severe blow.

*Treatment*—Immediate application of Ultra-Sound then ice.

Follow with general treatment rules. This injury is very slow in responding to treatment.

*Taping Method*—Athlete standing, leaning toward injury. Use 2-inch tape and place vertical strips (dotted lines) approximately 6 inches above and below the injury (Figure 37). Do not completely cover the buttocks as it will interfere with the motion of the thigh. Diagonal strips are then placed over the vertical strips. Horizontal strips can then be placed over the diagonal strips if you wish. Anchor the tape with an elastic figure-eight bandage as used in groin strain.

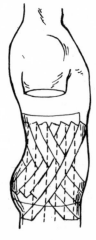

FIGURE 37. Taping for hip pointer.

*Doctor's Recommendation*—Steroids, Enzymes, Local Anesthetic, Skeletal Muscle Relaxants.

*Protective Equipment*—Crest of Ilium Pad; Peel Blocker (Figure 39).

LOW BACK STRAIN (*Sacro-Iliac*)

Pain in lumbo-sacral area, sacro-iliac area or perhaps in region of 11-12 thoracic vertebrae. Pain may go down back of leg.

*Cause*—Lifting a heavy object improperly, sleeping on a soft bed, a twisting fall, lifting and bending.

*Diagnostic Procedures*—(1) Bend sidewards, back muscles on affected side will remain in spasm. (2) Trunk-bending limited. Have to bend from hips, keeping spine rigid. (3) To diagnose side of low back pain, patient on back, trainer grasps under both of his flexed knees and lifts legs, swings raised hips from side to side; pain should develop. (4) To diagnose side of sacro-iliac sprain, patient on back and legs extended. Keeping knee straight, flex one leg at hip. Flexion will be limited on side of sprain.

*Treatment*—Sleep on a Board Bed; alternate whirlpool, microtherm, sound and Cramergesic Packs; back brace (Figure 39).

*Taping Method* (Figure 38)—Bend slightly forward with heels together and toes at a 45-degree angle. Using a basket-weave technique (dotted lines) alternate several strips of 2-inch tape from the buttocks angling up and across the back. Then, starting at the buttocks with horizontal strips overlap one another and extend up the back. For a sacro-iliac, a felt pad placed under the above tape may give additional relief. Apply a 4-inch elastic bandage over the tape.

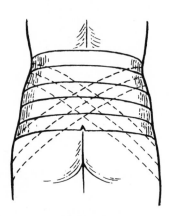

FIGURE 38. Taping for low back strain.

*Doctor's Recommendations*—Skeletal Muscle Relaxants, Enzymes, Local Anesthetics.

*Stretching Exercises*—Chapter XV

1. Number 3 and Number 4 under Diagnostic Procedure.
2. Figure 35 and #4 (Patients stretch under groin strains).

3. On back—trainer grasps ankle and flexes leg until knee almost touches stomach. Rotate knee in wide inward and outward circles.

4. Same as 3, only work with forearm under both knees, knees to chest and rotate.

5. On stomach—trainer reaches across the table and places hand on groin and lifts up; at same time, other hand below far shoulder blade with downward pressure.

6. On back—knees bent and feet close to buttocks. Bring right knee up to left shoulder and back to starting position. Repeat 12 times with each leg.

7. On back—leg on involved side flexed as far as possible and then suddenly extended.

8. On back or standing—pull in stomach and buttocks (gluteus) muscles and tighten them as if you were holding a dime between the buttocks. Throw hips forward (roll hips under).

## Low Back Bruise

*Treatment*—Follow general treatment rules, alternating moist heat and microtherm with Ultra-Sound and massage. Cramergesic Packs between treatments. Taping and doctor's recommendations same as for low back strain.

*Protective Equipment*—Cosby EK Back Pad, Back Brace (Figure 39).

## Fibrositis (*Lumbago*)

Fibrositis is an inflammation of connective tissue, muscle fibers, muscle sheaths, etc., often traced to bad teeth. There is usually formed in the area a soft swelling or knot which presses on nerves and causes pain. It can occur anywhere in the body where there are muscles. Most common site is between the shoulder blades (called fibrositis) but when it occurs in the lumbar region, it is called lumbago. It is also a common cause of stiff neck.

*Treatment*—Heat, Massage, Ultra-Sound and Steam Bath.

*Doctor's Recommendation*—Skeletal Muscle Relaxants, Enzymes, Local Anesthetics.

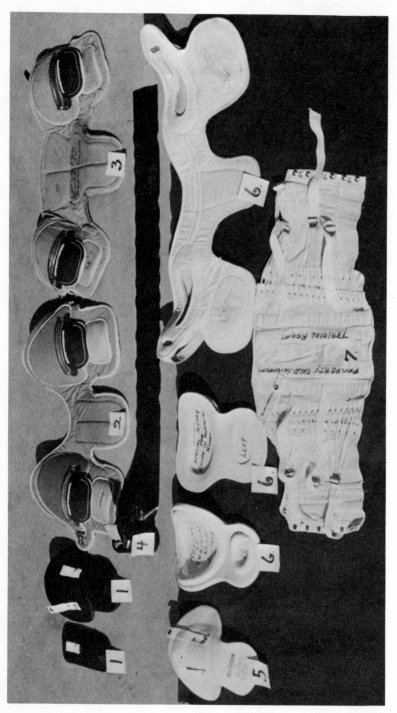

FIGURE 39. Protective equipment—Groin, Pelvis, Buttocks and Back.

1. Tail piece and hip pad
2. Hip injury pad
3. Low back injury pad
4. Rubber sling shot bandage
5. Hip pad
6. Pads for protection of a bruised hip
7. Back brace

## TRANSVERSE PROCESS

Projects from either side of each vertebra, a muscle attachment. It may be bruised, broken or muscles may be pulled from their attachment.

*Recognition*—Pain and muscle spasm in the area (similar to low back strain) with a possible shooting pain down the back of the leg. Is definitely an injury that should be taken care of by the team physician.

*Taping and Protective Equipment*—Same as for Low Back Strain.

## SLIPPED DISC

*Recognition*—An elastic disc of cartilage located between each vertebra. Injury usually occurs between the third, fourth, or fifth lumbar vertebra. The symptoms are: similar to acute sacro-iliac sprain; sciatic neuritis (aching, gnawing pain along course of nerve—back of leg); tingling, numbness of leg, foot and toes; foot drop; pain outside of lower leg (knee to calf) Figure 40.

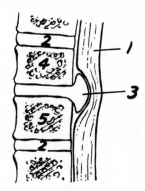

FIGURE 40. Normal and Abnormal Intervertebral Discs. (1) Spinal cord and nerve roots. (2) Normal intervertebral discs. (3) Disc has been ruptured into spinal cord, causing pressure on the nerves, etc. (4-5) Fourth and Fifth lumbar vertebrae.

*Treatment*—Definitely a problem for the team physician, X-ray, traction, surgery or he may suggest microtherm, whirlpool, Ultra-sound, manipulation and rehabilitative exercises (Chapter XV).

*Taping*—Same as Low Back Strain or use of a back corset (Figure 39).

BROKEN BACK

If in doubt or patient unconscious, call the team physician immediately. Treat as a broken neck if not sure (Chapter XIII). If both back and neck are broken, treat as a broken neck. If insufficient help or material is not available to move the patient or if you are not sure, cover him with a blanket and wait for adequate help. It is better to do nothing than to do harm.

*Recognition*—If patient is conscious, ask questions; he may complain of severe pain along his spine (tenderness, deformity); he may complain of inability to move some part of his body; injury to spine may result in paralysis of body below the point of injury (if he can move his fingers, but not his feet or toes, suspect a broken back); have him follow your finger with his eyes.

*Transportation*—The patient should be moved with the least rotation of his body as possible for fear of creating or causing additional neurological damage. In other words, place him on the stretcher in a position as nearly as possibly to the position in which he was found. If it is necessary to change the patient's position (vomiting, etc.) he should be transported lying on his stomach.

In placing a patient on a stretcher one should have at least three persons to help and you should not start until everyone knows what he is going to do. Place the stretcher as close to the patient as possible, with one person holding the patient's head, another his shoulders, and another his hips. At a prearranged signal gently lift the patient so the stretcher can be slid under him or if insufficient help is not available, lift him onto the stretcher.

If the patient is on his back and it is necessary to place him on his stomach, raise the arm on the side next to the stretcher. Kneel along stretcher opposite patient (one supporting head), grasp his clothing on far side and roll him slowly onto the board, face down. Strap patient to the stretcher and remain with him until he is turned over to the doctor (stretcher bearers should not be in step).

# CHAPTER XII

# Abdomen and Chest

## WIND KNOCKED OUT

*Recognition*—Often referred to as a blow to the Solar Plexus. Patient is on the ground, unable to breathe or talk and often making weird sounds in attempting to breathe.

*Treatment*—Patient on back; attempt to determine if any vertebra or rib injury; check his mouth for foreign objects or to see whether he has swallowed his tongue (Chapter XIII). With patient flat on his back, grasp his ankles and gently press the knees into the abdomen. Extend slowly and repeat (no pressure on rib cage or vertebrae) or apply artificial respiration by placing thumbs just below the rib cage (no pressure on rib cage or vertebrae), or in severe cases, use artificial respiration (Chapter XVIII). Do not at any time lift him by his belt or at the hips as this may add to the injury.

## STITCH IN SIDE

*Recognition*—Can occur in any athlete, but usually found among track and basketball players. Onset is usually quite rapid. Extreme pain usually in right side (stomach, ascending colon, and diaphragm).

*Cause and Prevention*—There are many theories, some are as follows: not in shape; constipation; accumulation of intestinal gases; salt deficiency; chronic; eating too much and too fast; greasy food; stomach, liver, gall bladder are supported by small muscles and ligaments—if overloaded with food or bile they go into spasms; internal organs (viscera) in some people are loosely supported and swing when they run, which causes the stitch; Doctors Crankshaw and Long (Australia) stated that "the stitch is associated with faulty, irregular breathing and does not occur in well-trained athletes."

*Treatment*—Eliminate the cause, slowly flex the right leg back to the abdomen, twist and stretch the stitch area, rest, relax, mild laxative, effervescent granules, wear a wide band supporter while competing, abdominal exercises (Chapter XV).

## SPLEEN

*Recognition*—The spleen is located in the upper left corner of the abdomen, toward the back (side), just below the diaphragm and in the region of the ninth to eleventh ribs. Its main function in so far as athletics is concerned is the storage of blood. An injury is usually caused by a crushing blow, a fall or a faulty block. The immediate reaction is usually mild shock, tenderness and local pain. In severe injuries, there is usually a pain in the left shoulder which runs about one third of the way down the arm along with shallow thoracic breathing. These symptoms may appear immediately or anywhere from an hour to days after an injury. This is called a delayed hemorrhage. If there is any doubt in your mind, or if the athlete has any of the above symptoms, *rush* him to the hospital.

## KIDNEY

*Recognition*—The kidneys are located on both sides of the spine and are partly covered by the last rib (from 11th thoracic vertabra to third lumbar). The left is slightly higher in the body than the right and both are approximately four inches long, two and one half inches wide and one inch thick. They can be injured by any type of a blow and will cause pain, tenderness, muscle spasms in the area, shock, nausea, vomiting and possibly internal bleeding and blood in urine.

In the event of any kidney or back injury, the individual should empty his bladder into a bottle the first two or more times after the injury. If there is any doubt in your mind, or if any of the above symptoms appear, the athlete should be taken to the team physician immediately.

## SHINGLES

*Recognition*—A very small, itching burning blister or "bleb" which usually starts on the nerve roots of the abdomen or side. The "blebs" fill with clear fluid first which later becomes cloudy.

*Cause*—The belief is that it is an infectious disease of virus origin (like measles or chicken pox). Contributing factors are: exhaustion, overwork, undernourishment, focal infection, emotions, fever, blood stream infections, etc.

*Treatment*—Use a cleansing drying preparation (Calamine, Ivy Dry, etc.) and a light covering; ultra-violet light; microtherm; paint with collodion. Doctors from time to time will prescribe Cortisone, gamma globulin, ACTH.

## RIBS—BROKEN, TORN CARTILAGE OR TORN MUSCLES

*Recognition*—This injury is usually due to a blow or a twisting or stretching of the area (wrestling). These injuries are painful but seldom serious unless the lung is punctured (rare), or the injury is in the region of the spleen. The injury can be recognized by pain (on movement, coughing, sneezing, deep breath); tenderness; crepitation; or the trainer can exert gentle pressure with one hand several inches in front of the injury and the other several inches behind the injury—gently pushing the ribs together—patient may be able to feel some crepitation, (either cartilage or bone) or a sharp, stabbing sensation; or have the athlete take a deep breath while the trainer applies gentle hand pressure over the area of the injury. This should relieve the pain. If there is any doubt in your mind about the injury, send him to the team physician.

*Treatment*—General treatment rules with emphasis on microtherm, ultra-sound and hot packs (Cramergesic).

*Taping*—Ribs are a problem to tape as it is impossible to absolutely immobilize them. Also, because of the continual movement of the rib cage, the patient often suffers tape burns. Because of the above we have been using a six-inch rib belt (Figure 49) on most of our rib injuries. There are, however, times when it is necessary (wrestling competition, etc.) to tape the rib and when this occasion comes up we use the following method: (Figure 41). Have the athlete stand with arm raised

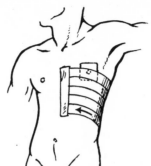

FIGURE 41. Taping ribs.

and hand resting on top of head. Anchor two-inch tape at the spinal column well below the injury. Have the athlete exhale completely then pull the tape around (following contour of ribs) and across to the center of the front of the body. Repeat above (overlapping tape) until the entire injured area is covered. Cover the nipple with a gauze pad. If the boy is going into competition, it may be necessary to lightly encircle the rib cage with three-inch elastic adhesive tape to keep the two-inch strips from loosening and peeling. If the injury is a torn rib cartilage place a piece of felt over the injury before taping. This will keep the cartilage in place.

*Protective Equipment*—Rib pads for protection; rib belt (Figure 49) in place of tape.

### BREAST BONE BRUISE OR SEPARATION

*Recognition*—The breast bone is technically known as the sternum and is divided into three parts: manubrium, gladiolus (or body), and the xiphoid process. Any part of this bone can be bruised and, on rare occasions, the manubrium is separated from the gladiolus. The injury is recognized by pain, swelling, tenderness, deformity, or crepitation. Send to team physician if you have any doubt about the injury.

*Treatment*—Relieve the pain and tenderness with microtherm, ultra-sound, etc. May also use a six-inch rib belt with a felt pressure pad under the belt and over the injury.

*Taping*—Similar to strapping for a sterno-clavicular sprain (Figure 41) only continue the basketweave down over the breast bone and add parallel strips to the basketweave starting at top of sternum and running toward the xiphoid process. A felt pressure pad over the area of the injury if there is a bone separation.

*Protective Equipment*—Special homemade pad to relieve pressure while playing (Figure 49); rib belt (Figure 49); sternum pad; and in some cases a clavicle splint will give relief.

STERNOCLAVICULAR SPRAIN

*Recognition*—This injury is commonly known as a separation of the collar bone from its attachments to the breast bone. This injury rarely occurs in mature athletes. It is more common in high school athletes. It is recognized by tenderness, swelling, deformity, and limited use of the shoulder.

*Cause*—Falling on the shoulder with a backward rotation, especially the tip of the shoulder; shoulder twisted backwards as in wrestling.

*Treatment*—Put arm in sling and send to team physician; General Treatment Rules.

*Taping*—Place a felt pressure pad over the joint and tape it as illustrated in Figure 42. Cover the nipple before taping.

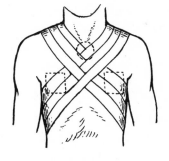

FIGURE 42. Taping for sterno-clavicular sprain.

*Protective Equipment*—Wear Big Boy, Jumbo or Line Backer Shoulder Pads or double Cantilever shoulder pads (Figure 47) to take the strain off this joint.

# CHAPTER XIII

# Neck, Face and Head

### NECK—STRAIN OR SPRAIN

*Recognition*—Usually in the trapezius muscle characterized by pain or stiffness. If pain is along cervical spine, treat as a broken neck.

*Cause*—A twisting or stretching of the neck muscles; sleeping with neck in a cramped position; a blow sharply snapping the head to the side.

*Treatment*—Ultra-sound; microtherm; medcollator, massage, standing in hot shower, hot packs in between other treatments. Traction and stretching exercises (not pops of vertebrae) as follows:

1.  On Stomach—head on soft pillow, turned to right. Trainer reverses hands (right hand on edge of right shoulder blade and left hand on head). Head held stationary and the pressure is only on shoulder and that is down and not out.

2.  On back—with head over edge of table and resting on trainer's knees, place one hand on patient's chin and other on his head. Head and neck in a straight line. Put head slowly through the following movements:

    a.  Turn head to left and then to right as far as you can.
    b.  Bend head to right and then to left.
    c.  Force head to chest as far as you can.
    d.  Force head back as far as you can.

3.  Standing position. Alternate single shoulder shrugging, then shrug both shoulders together.

4. Patient sitting or lying down and offering resistance to the following movements:

    a. Head back as far as it will go and trainer slowly forces it to chest against resistance.

    b. Head ¼ turn right and turn straight ahead against resistance. Same with head starting ¼ turn to left.

    c. Chin on chest and trainer slowly forces it to normal position.

    d. Same as b. only start with head flexed ¼ right and left.

*Taping*—We do not tape this type injury. However, some trainers have had success with the following method. Player sitting on a stool with shoulders thrown back. With 1½-inch adhesive, start with horizontal strips at hair line and continue to bottom of shoulder blade (extend out to lateral edge of shoulder blade). Next, apply 2-inch diagonal overlapping strips starting above nipples and pulling diagonally across shoulder (near neck) and down back attaching below shoulder blade on opposite side. Repeat procedure, forming an "x" at spinal column.

*Doctor's Recommendation*—Skeletal Muscle Relaxants.

*Protective Equipment*—A homemade collar (made out of sponge rubber and felt) or a rolled towel (Figure 44).

*Specific Exercises*—Chapter XV.

NERVE INJURY TO NECK

*Recognition*—Very often there is an injury to the neck and shoulder that leaves the characteristics of a nerve injury, numb with pins and needles or a burning sensation running down the arm to the fingers (similar to hitting the crazy bone). In all probabilities, the individual has injured the brachial plexus which arises from approximately the fourth to seventh cervical vertebrae and the first thoracic vertebra and is responsible for the nerve supply to the arm and hand.

*Cause*—A blow or twist that sharply snaps the head forward, backward or sideward.

*Treatment*—Gently pull (traction), shake and rotate the arm; massage the arm, neck and shoulders; traction to the neck; vitamin B¹; plus all of the treatment discussed under Neck Strain and Sprain.

*Taping*—Fold a towel (Figure 44) and tape it snugly around the neck. This will keep the head from being sharply snapped in any direction and thus eliminate the pressure on the brachial plexus. Instead of using a towel, one can use a collar made out of felt covered with sponge rubber and encased in stockinette. The stockinette can be tied, thus eliminating the tape or a shoe string can be placed through the center of the felt and laced into the shoulder pads to hold the collar in place. Another method to eliminate lateral flexion is to cut a ½-inch felt pad and fit it from tip of shoulder to the angle of the jaw. Secure this pad against the neck and shoulder with diagonal basketweave taping.

*Doctor's Recommendation. Specific Exercises*—Same as for Neck Strain.

### Broken Neck

Read article on Broken Back, Chapter XI.

*Recognition*—Patient should be treated as having a broken neck if he cannot open and close his fingers rapidly; if he cannot grasp your hand firmly; if he cannot, follow the movement of your finger with his eyes; if he does not show reflexes when hand is pricked with a pin (used if unconscious). If patient is unconscious, treat him as having a broken neck.

*Transportation*—The patient should be moved with the least rotation of his body as possible for fear of creating or causing additional neurological damage. In other words, place him on the stretcher in a position as nearly as possible to the position in which he was found. If it is necessary to change the patient's position he should be transported lying on his back. However, if he is vomiting, he may have to be turned on his side or stomach. When moving apply gentle traction to his neck and keep his head and neck in the same plane as his shoulders.

In placing the patient on a stretcher one should have at least three persons to help, and you should not start until everyone knows what he is going to do. Place the stretcher as close to the patient as possible. Assign one person to do nothing but apply gentle traction to his neck and keep his head and neck in the same plane as his shoulders; assign one person to the shoulders and one person to the hips and legs. At a pre-arranged signal, gently lift the patient just enough so the stretcher can be slid under him, or if sufficient help is not available, he can be lifted onto it. The entire body must be moved as a unit.

If the patient is on his stomach and must be changed, use a coordinated lifting roll as close as possible to the method described above when the patient was on his back, with one person definitely in charge of the neck and head.

When the patient is on the stretcher do not place anything under his head if he is on his back; if on side keep head and neck on same plane as the shoulders. Place sand bag, rolled newspapers, bricks rolled in a sweater, etc. on each side of the head to keep it from moving. Fold his arms over his chest and secure him firmly to the stretcher with anything you have that can be used to tie him down. Someone should guard his head and apply light traction during the entire trip to the hospital (stretcher bearers should not be in step).

## TEETH

Injuries to the teeth have always been a serious problem. With the advent of the face guard (Figure 44) and especially the individually fitted mouth-piece such as the Featherbite (Figure 43), our dental injuries have decreased tremendously. If a tooth is damaged, one should not apply digital pressure to test its looseness. See the dentist as soon as possible. The drinking of cold water or inhaling of cool air causes extreme pain if the nerve is exposed. Relief can be obtained by using oil of cloves and rubbing the outside of the cheek with ice.

If you wish to place a temporary cap on a tooth, dry the tooth thoroughly and then mold some warm dental wax, paraffin, beeswax, or candle wax over and around stump of the tooth. Another method is to chew two to three aspirins in some chewing gum and use this to cap the injured tooth. (Keep away from gums and do not leave on over two hours).

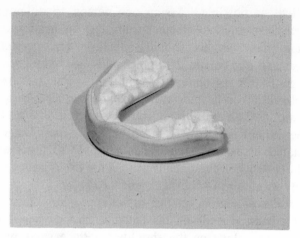

FIGURE 43. Featherbite mouth-piece.

### CHAPPED LIPS

Get out of the habit of moistening the lips with the tongue. Apply vaseline, inhalant, zinc oxide, or vitamin A and D ointment.

### COLD SORES

The feeling by many is that a cold sore is a virus infection. In so far as treatment is concerned, I have been having my best success with the application of Tuf Skin. This forms a protective covering and keeps out air and moisture. Other treatments are: Ultra-violet light, effervescing granules, vitamin A and D ointment, and Bacitracin.

### CUTS—MOUTH, TONGUE OR LIP

Saturate a piece of gauze with Nitrotan and keep on wound with direct pressure for 30 minutes. Consult the team physician in case the area needs to be stitched.

Usually heals quite fast. Be careful a food particle does not get into the wound. Use a mouthwash after each meal.

### DRY MOUTH

Usually due to nervousness, breathing through the mouth or drinking of milk prior to practice.

*Treatment*—Spray Spirits of Peppermint into the mouth; place

Cramergesic Balm (about size of small pea) on roof of mouth; Ascorbic Acid Lozenges; rub glycerine on inside of mouth; eliminate milk except at evening meal.

## PYORRHEA

Recognition—A chronic discharge of pus from the gums. In later stages, the gums become spongy and bleed easily. A problem for the dentist.

*Treatment*—Eat fresh salads and fruits, and use a toothbrush regularly. Use an antiseptic mouth wash (Hydrogen Peroxide if bad, in later stages one part Peroxide to one part water or a salt solution). Vince Tooth Powder (Sodium perborate) may be prescribed by the physician, usually used three times per day for one week, then one day a week. Vitamin C tablets.

## TRENCH MOUTH

*Recognition*—Any of the symptoms of Pyorrhea plus red inflamed gums. Highly contagious.

*Treatment*—Same as Pyorrhea. In addition, strict cleanliness must be observed with all eating or drinking utensils. The physician may also prescribe antibiotics.

## DISLOCATED JAW

*Recognition*—Cannot close mouth, and there is a dull ache just in front of the ears. Usually either one or both sides of the jaw will dislocate (forward). Jaw may be fractured.

*Cause*—A blow to chin while mouth is open; yawning; attempting to take too big a bite at one time.

*Treatment*—Wrap both thumbs and place in mouth on last two lower molars, fingers hooked under jaw. Press back and down with thumbs while pulling forward and upward (tilting) with fingers. As the jaw starts to return to its normal position, slip the thumbs out of the way to keep from getting bitten. It may not be possible to reduce a dislocated jaw without an anesthetic to relax the muscles. After reduction, immobilize jaw in a four-tailed bandage and send patient to team physician.

*Protective Equipment*—Face guard; rubber mouthpiece (Figure 43-44).

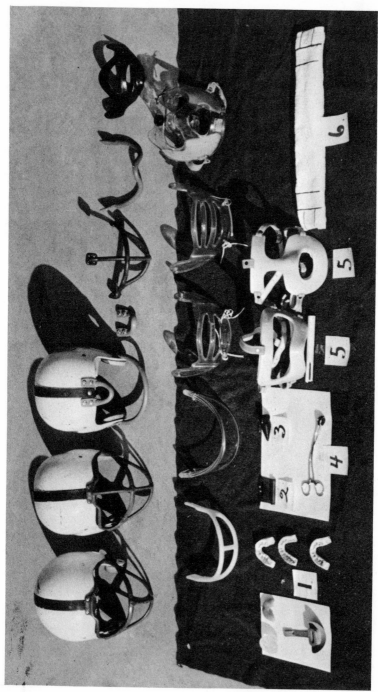

FIGURE 44. Neck, Face and Head. Upper two rows illustrates different types of football face protection.

1. Mouthpiece
2. Headgear snubber-protect bridge of nose
3. Oral screw
4. Tongue forceps
5. Face guards for sports other than football
6. Rolled towel

## FRACTURED JAW

Fractures of the jaw or cheek bone are very difficult problems and require the services of an oral surgeon.

*Recognition*—Movement of the jaw is painful, limited and teeth may not line up evenly.

*Treatment*—Gently close the jaw so teeth touch normally. Apply a four-tailed bandage and send to an oral surgeon.

*Food*—Malts (with or without eggs); concentrated baby food; mashed potatoes and vegetables; vitamins and various types of food that can be prepared in a blender.

## LOCKED JAW—TEETH

*Cause*—Blow to the face, blow to the solar plexus, or a muscular spasm.

*Treatment*—Be sure patient's neck is o.k.; if he is breathing normally, put him on his stomach which will aid him to relax and thus open his jaws; massage the jaw from in front of ears to chin; oral screw (Figure 44).

## SWALLOWING OF TONGUE

*Cause*—Same as locked teeth.

*Treatment*—If teeth are not locked, reach in and pull tongue forward with the finger or grasp it with a pair of tongue forceps (Figure 44). The tongue once pulled forward may "flip" back again. If so, once it is forward, hold it down with a tongue depressor, side of a pair of scissors, stick, etc.

If the teeth are locked, follow the treatment for locked jaw-teeth. As a last resort, (Figure 44), force the teeth open with an oral screw and then treat for the swallowed tongue.

## NOSE BLEED

*Prevention*—Wear a face mask while in competition.

*Treatment*—Place patient in a semi-reclining position; apply firm finger pressure on upper lip; cold towels or ice to nose, forehead and back of neck; pack nose with tampax or cotton saturated in adrenalin chloride, nitrotan or hydrogen peroxide; or pack with Nu Gauze Nose Pak. Do not permit athlete to blow his nose. If nose continues to bleed, send to team physician.

### BROKEN NOSE

*Recognition*—Deformity; gently move area back and forth and feel for crepitation; usually cartilage is broken away from the bone.

*Treatment—To Set*—Place thumbs on each side of the nose and with firm, light downward pressure (to relax and separate the cartilage away from the bone) gently ease back into position. Place tampax in each nostril and a gauze roll along outside of each nostril and tape to hold in place. Send to team physician and until completely healed, wear a "bird cage" face protector (Figure 44).

### FACE AND CHEEK BURNS

Some individuals (especially those with high cheek bones, prominent noses, etc.) have a tendency to have the skin rubbed off their faces. To prevent this, have them rub vaseline well into their skin before every practice and game. Protection (Figure 44).

### BRUISED EYE

*Cause*—A rupturing of the capillaries and small veins around the eye.

*Treatment*—Apply ice packs; do not blow nose as it may cause the eye to swell very rapidly. If so, suspect a fracture and send to a physician. Wear a "bird cage" face protector (Figure 44).

*Doctor's Recommendation*—Enzymes.

### FOREIGN BODY IN EYE

A foreign body in the eye is quite common. Sometimes, it is possible to remove or relieve the situation. If not, or in doubt, or if it feels as if it is still there, send the athlete to the team physician immediately; (patch over eye).

## DIRT, BUGS, ETC. IN EYE

If under the lower lid, it is usually easily seen and easily removed. Wipe it off with a piece of moistened sterile gauze or cotton applicator. If under the upper lid, draw the upper lid down over the lower lid and moisture produced by the eye may tend to make it stick on lower lid, or have patient look down; grasp eyelashes and gently roll the lid up with a match stick, etc. so the inside turns out. After removal of the object wash eye with Collyrium with Ephedrine, Visine, or a Boric Acid Solution.

## SCRATCH IN EYE

Should be treated by the team physician. Relief may be obtained from: Spectrocin Ophthalmic Ointment, 1% Yellow Mercuric Oxide Ophthalmic Ointment, Visine, Collyrium, Boric Acid Solution.

## STYE

Is usually an infection at the root of an eyelash and should be treated by the team physician. To bring the stye to a head, apply warm to hot wet dressings. Relief may also be obtained by using any of the preparations discussed under eye scratch.

## LIME IN EYE

Not as prevelant as in past years as most schools are now using other preparations to mark their fields. In the event of a lime burn, flush the eyes with a Boric Acid Solution, Crammers Eye Wash, or two drops of Castor Oil and send the athlete immediately to the team physician.

## CUT AROUND EYE

*Treatment*—To stop bleeding until patient can be taken to physician: digital pressure over sterile gauze, Gelfoam, hydrogen peroxide, nitrotan or Adrenalin Chloride Compress, Hemo Pak, ice. To close the wound apply Q.D.A. or Ace Adherent to skin (to make tape stick) and apply a butterfly bandage (Figure 2) or send to physician for suturing. To seal the wound, apply a small amount of vaseline across the incision and then apply flexible collodion.

## CONTACT LENS

The lightweight, transparent plastic almost unbreakable contact lens has become very popular in recent years. The size has been reduced from that of a nickel to the size of a lead pencil. Some athletes prefer the larger type because they are not apt to jar out during a game, whereas others prefer the more popular smaller, contour corneal lens. Likewise, their wearing time has been increased from three to four hours to a full day or more. Today about 85 per cent of the people with vision defects can be fitted with contact lenses. In a survey of 59 colleges and universities, Dr. Herbert S. Player reported that in the 1957 season, 161 boys wore contact lenses in football, 63 in basketball and 91 in other sports.

## WAX IN EAR

Never try to dig or pick anything out of an ear as it will probably only be pushed farther back and perhaps even puncture the ear drum.

*Recognition*—Discomfort, deafness, roaring sound in the ear.

*Treatment*—Syringe ear with hydrogen peroxide. Drain out and follow with a half-and-half mixture of Sodium Bicarbonate and alcohol. Send to team physician.

## FOREIGN BODY IN EAR

Read first paragraph under Wax in Ear.

*Recognition*—Discomfort, could be an insect, etc.

*Treatment*—Put a few drops of mineral oil, baby oil or olive oil in the ear and let it remain for a few minutes while the head is turned to the side. Then, let the oil run out and perhaps the foreign body will come out with it. If a bug, use a light and it may crawl out. If not, send to team physician.

## EAR FUNGUS

*Recognition*—A burning, itching sensation. Very common with swimmers.

*Treatment*—Wash with Boric Acid and Alcohol Solution twice a day. Send to team physician.

## CAULIFLOWER EAR

*Recognition*—Is an ear deformed from an injury in which the fluid under the skin has solidified so as to suggest a cauliflower.

*Cause*—An irritation caused by a twisting and turning of the ear as in wrestling, or from a headgear that has been twisted while on one's head. From a blow to the ear (boxing). This causes a collection of fluid within the ear tissue which unless removed will form a cauliflower ear.

*Prevention*—Rub vaseline onto ears; wear a wrestling head gear.

*Treatment*—Application of a pressure bandage and ice. If fluid appears, have it aspirated (removal with a syringe and needle) by the team physician. Follow with:

1. Fit a piece of cotton or soft sponge rubber behind the ear. Place a soft piece of sponge or cotton over the ear and secure with an elastic bandage. Can be examined daily, but should be left on from three to five days.

2. Apply a cast to the ear by alternating flexible collodion and gauze, shaping each layer (four of each) to the ear. Keep the cast on ear for five to seven days until sweat and wax loosens it. Peel off carefully so as not to irritate the underlying tissues. Do not apply a cast while ear is still hemorrhaging.

## CONCUSSION

Concussion is merely a term applied to an unknown result of a blow to the head or lower jaw and this description is used until a more definite diagnosis can be made by the team physician. There is a mommentary period of unconsciousness resulting from the blow (usually less than five minutes and seldom more than ten minutes). Even in the case of the so-called mild concussion, medical advice is essential as a safeguard against development of complications. Repeated small concussions lead to chronic more severe concussions. Watch the individual for twenty-four hours. You may even wish to awaken him every two hours. A good rule to follow is that any boy who has a loss of consciousness for only a moment, should be taken out of the game for examination.

*Recognition*—Following are some symptoms of concussions: loss of consciousness, a temporary amnesia, disorientation (will not be able to answer all present-day questions—temporary condition), headache (if over 12 hours, have re-checked by physician), dizziness.

More serious symptoms are: dilated, fixed pupils (moving finger test); pupils do not react to light; unequal pupils; blurring or loss of one-half vision; loss of sensation in extremities, numbness; prolonged drowsiness, vomiting (especially if it persists or starts an hour after injury); convulsions; paralysis; clear fluid from nose or ear; bleeding from ear (an indication of a skull fracture); coma.

*Movement*—Check neck, mouth and spine. If any doubt about the type of injury, treat as a broken neck (move lying flat on back, face up).

*Treatment*—Should be left in the hands of the physician. Temporary first aid; make sure air passage is clear; do not remove his headgear, have patient remove it himself; cold water and ice to neck and face; do not use ammonia inhalant while unconscious (may cause a jerk of head); administer oxygen; treat for shock (Chapter XVI); take patient to a hospital (ambulance) or keep him quiet in a semi-dark room.

*Test to help determine if athlete should continue to participate:*

1. Rhomberg's Sign—Feet together, arms down at sides, eyes closed. If athlete's body starts to sway or if he loses his balance, do not permit him to play.
2. Eyes Closed—Hands and arms out to side. Have the individual put index fingers together in front of him.
3. Eyes Closed—Arms in front. Quickly try and touch tip of nose with index finger (watch eyes).

4. Eyes open or closed—Feet toe to heel and arms straight forward. Check balance.

*Preventive Measures:*

1. Do not permit an athlete to enter a game until all major signs of a concussion have disappeared.
2. Wear a rubber mouthpiece (Figure 43-44).
3. Wear the best helmet available. If it is a suspension type headgear, be sure it fits the athlete correctly. To determine this, have the athlete (1) put hands on top of headgear and exert pressure. If it fits properly, he will feel pressure on top of the head. (2) If suspension is too close to the head, he will feel pressure on forehead or around the sides of the head.

# CHAPTER XIV

# Shoulder, Arm, Elbow and Hand

### ACROMIO-CLAVICULAR (SHOULDER) SPRAIN

*Recognition*—This injury is often called an A-C separation or a knocked down shoulder (if chronic). It can be recognized by pain especially if pressure is applied over the A-C joint; irregularity of shoulder tip can have an appearance of a lump on top (Figure 45) or a dropping appearance. Other symptoms are

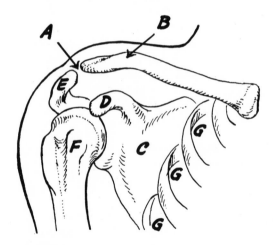

FIGURE 45. Front view of right shoulder.
A. Acromio-clavicular sprain—note displacement (hump) on top of outer edge of shoulder.
B. Clavicle (collar bone) where greatest number of fractures occur —at junction of two curvatures of the bone.
C. Scapula (shoulder blade).
D. Coracoid process of scapula.
E. Acromion process of scapula.
F. Humerus (ball of upper arm).
G. Ribs.

130

the ability to move the tip of the collar bone up and down, pain if arm is permitted to hang at side, especially if light traction is applied, loss of motion as demonstrated by following functional tests: (1) Athlete is unable to lift his arm to shoulder level. He cannot comb his hair. (2) He is unable to touch beyond the small of his back.

*Cause*—Falling on tip of shoulder, elbow, or hand with elbow locked, blow on top of shoulder, improper-fitting shoulder pads, muscles of shoulder not developed, arm tackle.

*Treatment*—Sling to support arm and elbow and refer to team physician. Observe treatment rules.

*Taping*—While shoulder is still in the acute state, exert upper pressure on the elbow to aid in reducing the separation. Keeping the shoulder in a semi-"shrugged" position (when shoulder is lowered, A-C joint will close) place a piece of felt 2 by 2 by ¼ in. directly over the joint. Secure the felt firmly with a strip of two-inch tape, starting on the chest and pulling up and over the shoulder and terminating on the lower edge of the shoulder blade. Remainder of taping is as illustrated in Figure 46 except we do not use elastic tape around the chest. In place of the elastic tape, secure the upper arm to the chest with an extra large rib belt (Figure 49). Finish by placing the arm in a sling. Remove for therapy when physician will permit. When physician will permit activity, strap the shoulder as illustrated in Figure 46, anchoring around the chest with 3-inch elastic adhesive tape (gauze pad over nipples before taping).

*Doctor's Recommendations*—Skeletal Muscle Relaxants, Steroids, Surgery.

*Protective Equipment*—All-Purpose Injury Pad (sponge) with hole cut to relieve pressure on joint (Figure 47); build up regular shoulder pads to relieve pressure; double Cantilever pad; Linebacker or Big Boy pads. All illustrated in Figure 47.

*Specific Exercises*—Chapter XV plus Figure 34 in Chapter XI and Figure 48.

BRUISED SHOULDER

*Recognition*—Any one of many muscles in the shoulder area may be bruised. However, it is usually the trapezius or the

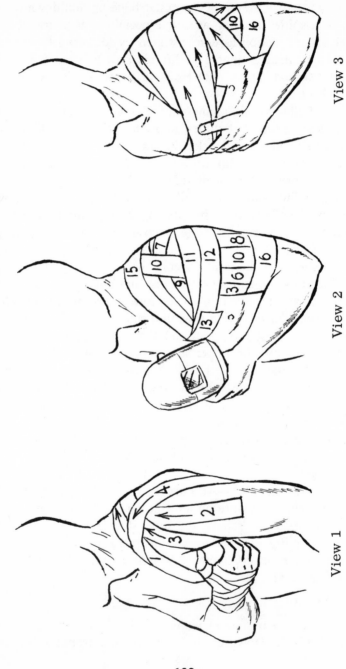

View 1          View 2          View 3

FIGURE 46. Steps in taping shoulder sprain, shown in three views, left to right.

132

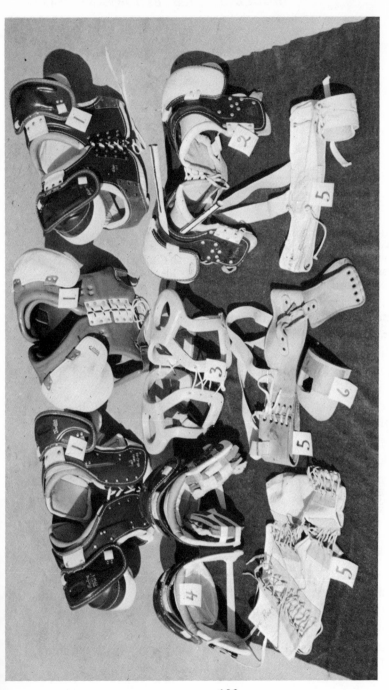

FIGURE 47. Shoulder, Arm, Elbow, Hand.

1. Heavy duty linebacker, big boy shoulder pads
2. Double cantilever shoulder pad (two rolls of paper denote the double cantilever)
3. Protection for under a shoulder pad
4. Home-made bruise pad—takes pressure off the shoulder
5. Shoulder harnesses (dislocations, strains and sprains)
6. All purpose injury pad with hole cut in top

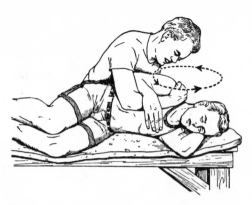

FIGURE 48. With many shoulder injuries, there is a tendency to hold the shoulder semi-rigid—favor it. As a result, unused tendons shorten, ligaments lose their elasticity and muscles develop adhesions—a step toward a "frozen shoulder." To prevent this, rotate the shoulder to the right and to the left as illustrated.

deltoid. These injuries are painful, but as a general rule, not serious and are characterized by the usual bruise pain and some functional disability.

*Cause*—Direct blow on top of muscle, improper-fitting shoulder pads.

*Treatment*—If necessary, support with a sling and follow general treatment rules.

*Taping*—Same as Figure 46 only place all-purpose sponge on shoulder with hole over bruise.

*Doctor's Recommendation, Protective Equipment and Specific Exercises*—Same as for acromio-clavicular sprain except no surgery.

### SHOULDER SPRAIN

The shoulder joint is held in place by a loose capsule supported by the tendons of subscapularis, supraspinatus, infraspinatus and the teres minor muscles, often referred to as the rotator cuff.

*Recognition*—Swelling, localized tenderness over the joint, loss of force and function, an arm-tackle shoulder.

*Cause*—Tendons over-stretched, (sometimes to the point of a tear) by a forcible twisting motion of the arm. Received in an arm tackle, blocking, and, quite often, in wrestling.

*Treatment and Taping*—Same as for chronic acromis-clavicular sprain (Figure 46), with special emphasis to assist the capsule or rotator cuff tendons (anchor tape above elbow and *pull* to neck). Likewise, secure upper arm to chest with a rib belt.

*Doctors' Recommendations, Protective Equipment and Special Exercises*—Same as for Bruised Shoulder.

## BURSITIS

*Recognition*—There are approximately 140 major bursae in the body. Three of these lie under the deltoid muscle at the tip of the shoulder (subdeltoid, subacromial, subcoracoid). Practically any injury to the shoulder involves a bursa, sometimes more severe than others. In many instances, it can become a chronic injury. In some cases, X-ray will reveal calcification in the injured tendon or bursa. The pain is very severe (often requires a strong analgesic and is especially prevalent when one tries to raise his arm above his head.

*Cause*—Friction, bruise, irritation.

*Treatment*—Should be under control of the team physician. Rest, Ultra-sound, microtherm, Cramergesic Pack, Massage above and below bursa.

*Doctor's Recommendation*—Steroids, Skeletal Muscle Relaxants. Surgery, Enzymes.

## SHOULDER DISLOCATION

*Recognition*—The shoulder is a ball-and-socket joint and a dislocation occurs when the humerus (ball) slips out of its junction in the glenoid fossa (socket in shoulder blade). It can dislocate forward (most common is when ball goes under coracoid process) or backward (ball under spine of scapula). The usual symptoms are: severe pain and tenderness over the area; a deformity of the shoulder—a hollow indentation where bone should be, and a prominent lump (head of humerus under armpit) where it should not be; loss of function; elbow is unable to touch side of body; cannot touch hand to opposite shoulder; severe muscle spasm around joint.

*Cause*—A blow while arm is bearing weight, a rotation such as a catcher throwing a ball to second base, a twisting of the joint (wrestling).

*Methods of Reduction*—In a forward dislocation, the head of the humerus is in a position to rupture the brachial artery, vein, and nerves. A trainer should attempt a reduction *only* if he has been taught the methods acceptable to his team physician and also has his permission to attempt the reduction. Immediate reduction, if permissable, is advantageous in that it will reduce the muscle spasm and will not stretch the capsule and ligaments in the joint. If the individual will not relax and if the muscles contract, it is not advisable to try to reduce a dislocation without giving the patient a sedative or an anesthetic.

1. Kocher Method—Patient seated: (a) elbow is gently brought in close to patient's side, forearm is at right angle and straight ahead; (b) holding the elbow in this position, rotate the forearm outward almost to a right angle to the body. (c) With forearm held in this position, the elbow is slowly and gently lifted to an angle of about 60 degrees; (d) forearm is quickly brought across in front of the body while the elbow is held in the raised position; (If an assistant is available have him place a towel under patient's armpit and lift slightly as you start section "c").

2. Prone Method—Patient on back: (a) trainer removes shoe and places his longitudinal arch in patient's armpit, and graps the injured's wrist with his hands; (b) exert a light, steady continuous pull on arm until muscles relax; (c) slowly carry arm toward patient's body with a slight inward rotation.

3. Mexican Method—Patient on back with arm out at right angles to body: (a) trainer removes shoe and places sole of his foot on patient's ribs just below armpit, and grasps wrist with both hands; (b) exert a slight pull on the wrist and at same time push the foot gently into the ribs.

If an individual has a chronic shoulder (dislocated three or more times), he will probably be able to reduce it himself. This type shoulder will probably have to be operated on.

*Treatment*—In full charge of team physician. Follow general instruction treatment rules. Rest, microtherm, massage and rehabilitative exercises.

*Taping*—Figure 46 with a 6-inch rib belt around upper arm and chest. Arm in a sling.

*Doctor's Recommendation*—X-ray, Surgery.

*Protective Equipment*—Shoulder harness to prevent raising of arm above 85 degrees; built-up shoulder pads, double cantilever pad, Linebacker or Big Boy pads. All illustrated in Figure 47.

Nerve Injuries to Shoulder (Chapter XIII)

Upper Arm Bruise—Myositis Ossificans

*Recognition*—A bruise (Charley horse if on thigh. See Chapter X) to the brachialis anterior muscle (front side of upper arm), right where the cap of the shoulder pad ends when arm is raised. The bruise may rupture the bone-covering (periosteum) and liberate bone-forming cells (osteoblasts) which begin to grow in the muscle. This condition is known as Myositis Ossificans which is a calcification in the muscle, and may occur in any muscle in the body. It is quite painful.

*Prevention*—Wear shoulder pads that fit properly. Have an extra-thick layer of padding attached to the cap which will protect the upper arm when contact is made.

*Treatment*—Same as Charley horse in Chapter X. If Myositis Ossificans develops, treatement should be under care of physician who will take periodic X-rays of the arm to note the development of the calcium deposit. (We have been having good luck with Ultra-sound.) It is usually two to three weeks before a shadow will appear on the X-ray film and, by five or six weeks, there will be evidence of bone formation. By the end of five or six months, the arm will be quite painful as a bursa has probably been formed between the new bone-deposit and the muscle (Bursitis).

It is not uncommon for the new bone-deposit to attach to the bone of the upper arm.

*Doctor's Recommendation*—Enzymes, Surgery (has been quite successful).

*Protective Equipment*—See prevention; make a protective cup out of castex or fiber glass and tape to arm; insert a fiber pad in a sponge rubber knee pad and wear on upper arm at all times (Figure 49).

### STRAINS AND HYPEREXTENSION OF ELBOW

*Recognition*—See tests for hyperextended knee in Chapter X. Flex elbow to 90 degrees and flex and extend fingers; pain will be felt in muscle attachments.

*Cause*—Falling on extended arm, elbow bent backwards, a twisting of the joint.

*Treatment*—Follow treatment rules.

*Taping*—Bend elbow from 15 to 45 degrees and tape same as for an over-extended knee (Chapter X).

*Doctor's Recommendation*—Steroids, Enzymes.

*Protective Equipment*—Hockey elbow pad (Figure 49). Foam rubber (plastic) padding.

*Specific Exercises*—Chapter XV.

### FLUID ON ELBOW

Same as treatment for fluid on knee (Chapter X). Same protective equipment as for Hyperextended Elbow.

### BONE CHIPS ON ELBOW

Work bone chips out of joint and treat as any bruise. Protect with hockey elbow pad (Figure 49) or foam rubber elbow pad. Surgery after the season is over.

### TENOSYNOVITIS—Refer to Chapter IX.

### TENNIS ELBOW—PITCHERS' ELBOW

*Recognition*—Dull or sharp pain over lateral condyle of

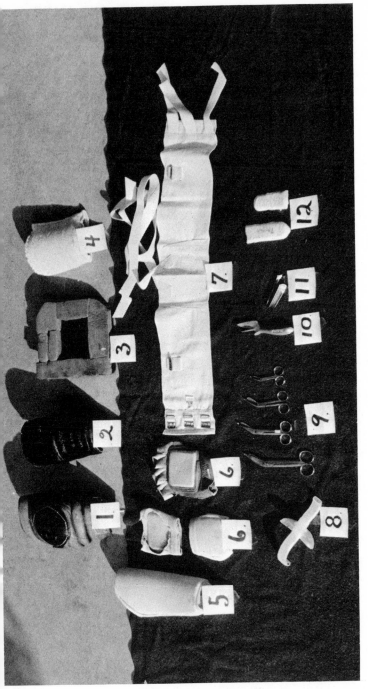

FIGURE 49. Shoulder, Arm, Elbow, Hand.

1. Elbow bruise pad
2. Fracture glove
3. Sternum or chest injury pad—lace to shoulder pads
4. Upper arm bruise pad—fiber and sponge rubber
5. Forearm pad
6. Hand pads
7. Rib belt
8. Resusitube Airway
9. Bandage Scissors
10. Tape cutter
11. Handle of a spoon made splint into a finger
12. Felt thumb pads

humerus; pain and weakness down forearm when lifting an object with forearm (palm down, pronation) and the elbow fully or partially extended. Pain is absent when lifting with palm up (supination). Individual may complain that condition feels like rheumatism in the arm and elbow.

*Cause*—Authorities do not agree as it is often found in baseball, golf, handball, tennis, etc. players as well as in painters, carpenters, welders, etc. One theory is that it is caused by a twisting motion when inadequately warmed up and thus affects the pronater teres muscle. Another theory is that it is caused by a forced rotation of the forearm (palm up and palm down) with elbow extended. It is not associated with a bruise, but is usually prevalent after activity.

*Treatment*—Splint elbow and wrist. Remove splint for daily therapy.

*Doctor's Recommendation*—Steroids, Enzymes, Surgery.

## DISLOCATED ELBOW

*Recognition*—Pain, deformity, inability to bend at joint. Usually a backward displacement of the ulna and radius (forearm) at elbow joint. Sometimes the radius only is dislocated and if so, this is forward.

*Cause*—A violent twist of the forearm; fall on the hand.

*Reduction*—Extremely difficult to set. Rarely possible without anesthesia. Never attempt to reduce without adequate medical aid except in a rare emergency. It is better to place the arm in a splint and take patient to a hospital and then help the physician with the reduction.

*Emergency Reduction*—Patient on back. Assistant holds patient's arm under armpit. Doctor will grasp wrist and gently pull the arm as he works the bone into place with the other hand.

*Treatment*—Pressure, ice, splint and take to physician. If arm is put in a cast forearm muscles can be exercised by gripping a ball until cast is removed.

*Doctor's Recommendation*—Steroids, Enzymes.

*Special Exercises*—Chapter XV.

## COLLES' FRACTURE

The most common type of forearm fracture is one at the lower end of the radius (in region of wrist, behind thumb) and is called a Colles' Fracture.

*Recognition*—Very often this injury is mistaken for a sprained wrist as it has the usual symptoms of a sprain. If pain, tenderness, or loss of motion in this area, the athlete's arm and wrist should be X-rayed.

*Cause*—Fall on extended hand in which the hand is forced backward and outward; severe blow (baseball), straight arm.

*Treatment*—Cast by physician.

*Taping*—As for a sprained wrist and hand, with additional sponge rubber padding over and around the injury.

*Protective Equipment*—Fracture Glove (Figure 49).

*Specific Exercises*—Chapter XV.

## WRIST INJURIES

The wrist is composed of eight carpal bones. It may be bruised, sprained, dislocated, or any one of the bones may be broken.

*Recognition*—In a bruise or sprain, the usual symptoms are tenderness, pain, deformity.

In a dislocated wrist, which is rather unusual, there is a strong resemblance to a Colles' Fracture. It should be placed in a splint, and the patient taken to the team physician. Treatment will resemble that of a Colles' Fracture.

In a broken wrist, the above symptoms hold true. Any one of the bones may be broken. However, it is usually the scaphoid (navicular) which is located in the hollow area between the base of the thumb (first metacarpal) trapezium (greater multangular) and the wrist in what is sometimes called the "snuff box." The scaphoid has a very poor blood supply and thus heals very slowly.

*Fracture Tests*—(1) Tap with finger or top of pencil on "snuff box" or over tender area. (2) Close fist and tap on end of knuckles. (3) Gently pull thumb and fingers.

*Treatment*—General Treatment rules. If any doubt, send to team physician.

*Taping*—The first rule in taping the wrist or hand is to spread the fingers so as to increase the size of the wrist which will reduce the possibility of applying the tape too tightly. Secondly, always tape over gauze to prevent friction, etc. There are many ways of taping the wrist, some are:

1. Wrist is encircled with three to five overlapping strips of 1½-inch adhesive tape.

2. Hand and wrist wrap (Figure 50). Using 1-inch tape,

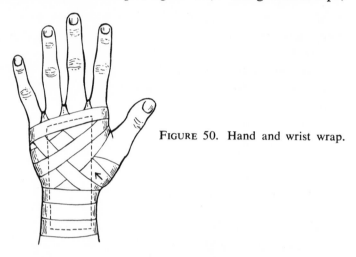

FIGURE 50. Hand and wrist wrap.

this wrap can be used to support a weak wrist and hand. To protect a bruised hand, a piece of sponge rubber one-half the size of the dotted line can be placed on the back of the hand, held in place with ½-inch tape placed between the fingers. For a sprained wrist (to prevent the wrist from bending forward), place a piece of ¼-inch felt on back of hand (dotted line). Anchor between the fingers and cover with a hand and wrist wrap.

3. To prevent wrist from bending forward, place four strips of 1½-inch tape from base of fingers to wrist. Fold ends of tape back to prevent from slipping. Cover with hand and wrist wrap.

4. To prevent wrist bending backward, place four strips of 1½-inch tape from base of fingers across palm to wrist. Cover with hand and wrist wrap.

5. One can use an ankle wrap in place of the one-inch tape in any of the above.

*Protective Equipment*—Fracture glove; Absorblo elastic protector (both in Figure 49). Boxing glove.

*Specific Exercises*—Chapter XV.

## HAND INJURIES

The hand as we usually refer to it consists of five metacarpal bones. These bones may be fractured or dislocated. Dislocations, however, are rather rare. The symptoms, treatment, taping, fracture tests (add crepitation test), protective equipment and exercises are as have been discussed under Wrist Injuries.

Often when the back of the hand (or foot) is bruised, a *blood vessel* is ruptured. This is evident by a quick, large-sized soft swelling. Follow the general treatment rules of immediate pressure and ice. For overnight treatment, place a piece of soft sponge rubber over the ruptured blood vessel, bandage wrist and hand with an elastic bandage and instruct the athlete to keep his hand elevated. Check for fracture.

## THUMB AND FINGERS

The thumb and fingers are made up of 14 phalanges bones. The surface of this area may suffer abrasions, bruises, or blood under the nail. These types of injuries have been discussed in previous chapters.

These bones may also be fractured or the joints dislocated or sprained.

*Fracture Tests*—Any of these bones may be fractured. Test the bone in the following manner to help determine if the bone is fractured:

1. Gently pull thumb or finger, light lateral movement feeling at all times for crepitation. 2. Tap with finger over tender area. 3. Tap on end of straight finger or thumb.

*Dislocation*—Joint is usually dislocated backward.

*Reduction of Dislocation*—Patient's palm down, hold finger firmly just below dislocation with one hand; grasp finger just above dislocation with other hand. Tip of thumb on "hump" of dislocation, index finger directly under dislocated joint. With index, second and third fingers grasping the injured finger, pull finger and at same time gently force the dislocated joint into position with the thumb.

*Treatment*—Follow treatment rules, then place in a splint (tongue depressors, metal, etc.) and have X-rayed. The following treatment is similar to the treatment of any sprain, with special emphasis on heat of any type to increase the usual poor circulation in this area. Also, the area should be exercised daily by grasping a rolled (4 by 5 by ½ inch) piece of sponge rubber.

*Taping*—There are many taping methods. I will illustrate a few (Figures 51-55). Any of these methods may be combined with any of the other methods.

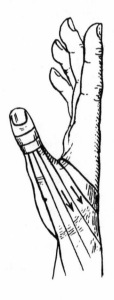

FIGURE 51. Taping for a sprained thumb. To prevent thumb from bending into palm apply ½" strips of tape from base of thumb-nail down back of thumb to wrist. Apply a figure eight basketweave (Figure 53) over the above. To prevent thumb from going backwards, apply ½" strips down inside of thumb to palm of hand and anchor with a figure eight basketweave. In place of tape strips, one can substitute a piece of ⅜" felt in either of the above (Figure 49).

*Doctor's Recomendations*—X-ray, Splint.

*Protective Equipment*—Fracture glove; hand bruise pads; end of tablespoon folded over to protect tip of finger and joint (Figure 49).

*Specific Exercises*—Chapter XV.

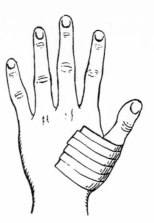

FIGURE 52. This is the first step in taping a badly sprained or dislocated thumb. Starting at base of thumb joint, apply several strips of one-inch tape from back of the hand to the palm. Cover with any other thumb-taping method (Figure 51 or Figure 53).

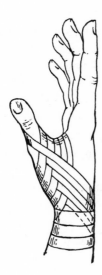

FIGURE 53. Figure 8 basketweave for a sprained or disclocated thumb.

FIGURE 54. Taping for a sprained thumb. Using ¾″ tape, apply it around the thumb and hand. Pinch the tape together between thumb and hand and reinforce with a short piece of tape. If desired, this taping may be carried around the thumb and index finger instead of around the entire hand.

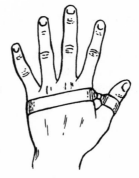

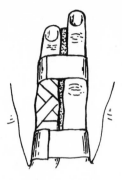

FIGURE 55. Taping for a sprained or dislocated finger. Flex the injured joint slightly. Using ½″ adhesive tape apply a basketweave over the injured joint. Place a ⅛″ thickness of soft sponge, felt or cotton between the fingers (optional) to prevent friction. With ½″ tape, tape to an adjoining finger which will act as a splint. Leave the index finger free if possible.

### BASEBALL FINGER

*Recogition*—This is a tearing of the extensor tendon from its insertion in the base of the distal phalanx of any finger (distal joint). Often referred to as a "dropped finger."

*Cause*—A blow on the tip of the finger which causes a forced flexion of the joint while the tendon is contracted.

*Treatment*—Place a roll of gauze bandage in the palm of the hand. This will keep the proximal interphalangeal joint in slight flexion and the distal (injured) joint n complete extension. Tape in place.

*Doctor's Recommendation*—X-ray, Splint.

*Protective Equipment*—Tablespoon, folded over to protect tip of finger and joint (Figure 49).

*Exercises*—Same as for thumb and fingers.

### CRACKED SKIN

*Recognition*—A peeling, cracking, hardening, drying of the skin.

*Cause*—Nerves, weather.

*Treatment*—Relax, vitamin A & D ointment, Glycerin, Mineral Oil, Foot Ointment (Cramer's), Toilet Lanolin.

# CHAPTER XV

# Rehabilitative Exercises of Specific Area Injuries

The rapidity of the rehabilitation of an injury is determined by one's desire. One must work to reach his goal. With true dedication, one can rehabilitate almost any injury. There is a great difference between wishing and accomplishing the desired goal. Between the two lies a lot of hard work, both physical and mental. *Remember that what you can do tomorrow depends on what you do today.*

In working with weights, one must remember that heavy resistance with low repetitions builds strength and high repetitions with light resistance builds endurance. Continue to add weights as lifting-power increases. See Dr. Brashear's comments on this in Chapter III.

When lifting weights, breathe deeply on lifting and exhale on lowering. There are numerous weight-lifting formulas. Some of the more popular are:

1. Lift maximum weight 30 times in three series of 10 lifts each with a two-second hold and a two-second rest between each lift. Rest two to three minutes between each series of ten.

2. Determine maximum weight and hold it as long as possible (knees). Do three to five times.

3. Weight formula. Determine the maximum weight you can lift (say it is 28 lbs.). Lift ½ of maximum weight (14 lbs.) ten times. Rest and lift ¾ of maximum weight (21 lbs.) ten times. Rest and lift full weight (28 lbs.) ten times.

4. Heavy-to-light formula. Determine maximum weight and lift ten times. Rest and then lift five lbs. less than maximum ten times. Rest and lift five lbs. less ten times. Example: 30 - 25 - 20.

Be sure there is an adequate warm-up before each exercise period—running, stretching, rope-skipping, etc.

### ARCH, ANKLE AND LOWER LEG EXERCISES

(Wear correctly-fitted shoes. Do not wear loafers, flats or thongs.)

1. On back or sitting. Extend foot as far as possible, pointing toes downward. Then flex foot as far as possible, point toes upward.

2. On back or sitting. Turn soles of feet inward so they face each other, then outward.

3. On back or sitting. Foot circumscribes small circle. Ball of foot down first, then in, then up.

4. On back or stomach. Start with soles of feet together, then breast-stroke kick.

5. Sitting, injured leg across opposite knee. Using hand forcibly flex, extend, invert, evert and rotate the foot and ankle.

6. Stand erect. Walk on outside of feet, toes curled in. Or walk on supination board (triangle board).

7. Stand with feet one foot apart and toeing in. Rise on toes as high as possible (without pain).

8. Stand erect, then rise as high as possible on heels.

9. Squat to one-half knee bend without raising heels from the floor.

10. Ankle Disc—round disc 14-inch diameter with ½ croquet ball screwed on the bottom. One foot near each edge of disc. Make disc run around its edge on the floor.

11. Rock up on toes and back again. Hold weights in hands to increase resistance.

12. Stand on outer edge of feet and roll them back to normal again.

13. Stand on outer edge of feet and then go up on toes.

14. Run barefoot in sand, forward, backward, zig-zag.

15. Run backwards.

16. Rope-jumping.

17. Walk naturally. Just before foot touches floor point foot inward (pigeon toe).

18. Calf-gripper. Bring foot up to knee and grip opposite calf with toes and arch.

19. Stand, sit, etc. Heels together and toes out, to toes together and heels out.

20. Duck-waddle. From ¼ to ½ knee bend position (never full knee bend).

21. Inchworm. Feet together and parallel, knees straight with heels and hands on floor. Series of short steps with hands. Heels on floor as long as possible, until the body is prone, then walk back to upright position.

22. Ride a bicycle everywhere you go (stay out of cars).

23. Stand erect, feet flat on floor. Force knees as far forward as possible, keeping heels on floor.

24. Stand 30 inches from wall; move body to wall keeping heels in contact with floor at all times.

25. Sit on chair. Tap heel then toe to floor, etc.

26. Place golf ball under foot and roll it from toe to heel, etc.

27. Pick up marble with toes. (a) Place in hand opposite knee of good leg. (b) Place in hand behind buttocks of injured leg.

28. Sitting position. Feet on towel. Pull towel up under foot with toes. May place a weight on end of towel to offer resistance.

29. Sitting position. Hold one leg straight and slowly bring opposite toe up shin as far as possible.

30. Roll sole of foot over coke bottle or baseball bat. Place toes on a book and rock heels to ground. Place heels on a book and rock toes to ground.

31. Using weights, invert, evert, flex, extend foot (also while in whirlpool).

32. Run or walk up steps on toes (stadium steps).

33. Stationary bicycle.

34. Swim.

KNEE EXERCISES

The knee is just as good as the quadriceps (thigh) muscle is strong. It forms the first line of defense against knee injuries, and when it is weakened, strain on the ligaments develop.

Knee injuries seldom occur unless the foot is firmly fixed to the ground. Injuries in the pile-up may be greatly reduced by keeping the knee flexed.

1. Exercises while confined to bed or cast:

   A. Flexor. Flex muscles of thigh and buttocks and draw knee cap toward pelvis. Hold until leg gets tired. Do anytime; in cast, class, movies, bull session, dinner, etc.

   B. Leg raising. With knee joint locked (either in cast or out), lift leg up (to right angle) and lower slowly. Two minutes every hour while in cast.

   C. Resistive leg raising. Same as above, only rest the ankle of the uninjured leg on the injured ankle and offer slight resistance to the raising of the injured leg.

*Continue all of the above exercises after cast has been removed.*

2. Limited Flexion Exercises:

   A. Sit on table with leg extended over edge. Weight of leg will gradually drop it into full flexion.

   B. Sit on table. Grasp shin and slowly pull to buttocks.

   C. Lying on abdomen, place bandage around foot and hold in both hands. Attempt to flex knee by pulling on bandage.

3. Limited Extension Exercises:

   A. Standing. Place heel of injured leg on a low chair and hands on knee (patella). Slowly force knee back (extension).

4. Lateral Leg-Swing. Place extended arm (laterally) opposite injured leg against wall. Swing injured leg out laterally, then across in front of leg as far as possible.

5. Gravity Swing. Sit on table and swing leg back and forth.

6. Resistive Drills (See first few paragraphs of this chapter).
   A. Sit on table and raise leg against gravity.
   B. Weights. Sit on table with weights on foot. Raise weights until leg is parallel to floor (execute in three series of ten and with two seconds between flexion and extension). Increase weights.
   C. Same as B only place maximum weight load on foot. Raise and hold just as long as possible (until quadriceps become tired). Rest and repeat three times.
   D. Pulley Weights. Flex and extend leg from sitting or lying position.
   E. Knee Press. Stand with feet apart, knees slightly flexed and hands on outside of knees. Press knees together with hands, knees offering resistance. Repeat outward.
   F. Wall Push. Stand erect one yard from wall and try to force foot through the wall, keeping leg straight.
   G. Bed Lift. Stand with your back to an unliftable object which is about two feet from the ground. Try lifting the object with the heel of the affected leg.
   H. Bar Press. On back with feet under bar (weights on end of bar. Push up as far as possible, and slowly let it back down.
7. Stadium Steps. "Jog" up steps, and walk down (can add weight by carrying a dummy).
8. Knee Bends. Grasp bars (stall) with hands and do a ¼ or ½ knee bend. (Do not use full knee bend or duck waddle.)
9. Running. Emphasize leg extension by snapping the lower leg forward with each stride.
10. Run backwards.
11. Walk up steps backwards.
12. Bicycle Riding (Buy an old bicycle and stay out of cars).
    A. Riding, with force coming from injured leg.
    B. Stationary bicycle.
    C. On back. Palm of hands under buttocks, leg straight and toes pointed.
    D. Same as C only add weights to foot.

13. Walk on toes. Can add weight by carrying dummy.

14. Raise weight high on toes up and down.

15. Heel-touch. Straddle position with arms over head. Right hand touch rear of left heel, etc.

16. Leg-swing. On back. Raise leg to perpendicular with knee straight then swing leg across body until toe touches floor on opposite side. Hip and shoulders remain on floor throughout.

17. Hurdle Spread. Sitting in hurdle spread position, with injured leg extended. Touch extended toe with opposite hand.

18. Quadriceps Builder. Sit on bench ¾ inch behind knees, toes under stall bars and trunk erect. Raise body by contracting quadriceps and straightening legs. Weight can be increased by backward lean of body.

19. Sit-Ups. Hook toes under stall bars. Sit up and touch right toe with left hand, and left toe with right hand.

20. Rocker. Flat on back. Raise legs to a perpendicular position, grasp toes and rock back and forth.

21. Circle Drill. On back with legs straight. Raise the injured leg (45 and then 90 degrees) and rotate it in small circles in both directions. Repeat with both legs.

22. Flutter Kick. On stomach with legs straight and knees semi-locked. Move the legs up and down in the same motion as the flutter kick in the pool.

23. Canvas Strap. Sitting position with a canvas strap (which is attached to wall or table) around calf of leg. From this position, stand up without using hands.

24. Rowing.

25. Swimming (crawl, not breast stroke).

In conclusion, always remember a well-developed quadriceps muscle is the best possible indication of a strong, healthy knee.

THIGH EXERCISES

1. Any of the knee or leg, hip, or low back exercises which stretch the thigh muscles.

2. Sit on a table and permit leg to swing like a pendulum.

3. Standing with legs spread and hands on groin, bend all four ways and rotate.

4. On knees with hands on groin, bend slowly backward.

5. Split position with left leg forward and right leg back (knee on ground). Support with hands on floor below forward thigh. Bounce gently up and down, then reverse legs.

## HAMSTRING EXERCISES

After each exercise, touch toes 10-12 times from a standing position as hamstring muscles have a tendency to shorten during activity.

1. Any of leg, hip, or low back exercises that stretch the hamstring muscles plus knee exercise numbers 1A, 3A, 4, 6F, 6G, 15, 16, 17, 20.

2. Feet apart, bend over and bounce.

3. Standing. Squat until thighs are parallel to floor and heels and hands on the floor. Raise buttocks with hands remaining on floor.

4. Sitting position. Grasp knees and pull to chin and then rock back and forth.

5. On back. Have team-mate slowly rotate leg and at same time, exert tension (pull).

6. On back. Trainer flexes knees as much as possible and at same time rotates knee in outward and inward circles.

7. Sit-ups. Elbow or forehead to opposite knee.

8. Stand with toes on end of a step (holding rail for balance) and then lower the heels as far as possible.

9. Cross the legs and then bend over and touch the toes with the fingers. Alternate the crossed legs.

10. Functional test Number One as explained in Chapter X.

11. On stomach or standing. With weights on the foot, flex the knee to just short of 90 degrees. Beyond 90 degrees hamstrings relax and lateral sway may develop. Read weight procedure at start of chapter.

## STRETCHING EXERCISES—UPPER LEG, GROIN, HIP, LOW BACK

All stretching exercises should be done slowly, no sudden jerks or speeding up.

1. All groin and back exercises in Chapter XI.

2. Sitting Semi-Split (Hips, Legs, Back, Crotch, Knees). Sitting. Spread legs as far as possible and grasp ankles. Keep knees straight and touch forehead to floor. Hold five seconds, relax and repeat.

3. Standing Semi-Split (Hips, Legs, Back, Crotch, Knees). Standing. Same as above only from standing position (pull downward, trying to touch head to floor). Hold five seconds, relax, and repeat.

4. Chest to Wall (Front Thigh). Stand facing wall with chest touching and feet close. Raise leg back and up. Grasp instep with hand and pull leg up as far as possible. Head back and knee must not be out to side. Hold for five seconds, relax, and repeat.

5. Knee Press (Buttocks, Hip and Back). Lie flat on back. Team-mate holds one leg down and presses opposite knee toward armpit. Stretch as far as possible, hold five seconds, relax, and repeat.

6. Table Sit (Hips, Crotch, Buttocks, Knees, Inside Thigh). Spread legs as far as possible. Hold back of table. Lower buttocks straight down and try to sit on floor. Bounce up and down, relax, and repeat.

7. Knees In (Hip, Knees). Sitting. Feet spread as far as possible with knees straight. Bend legs inward until knees touch. Try and touch the floor with inside of knees. Hold five seconds, relax, and repeat.

8. Inchworm (Hamstrings). Palms flat on floor, two feet in front of feet. Slowly straighten legs until knees are straight. Move hands in closer to feet. Hands and feet flat on floor at all times. Relax and repeat.

9. Hurdle Touch (Groin, Crotch, Inside Thigh). Place inside of knee on table or chair. Touch floor beside foot with both hands. Hold three seconds, bounce three times, relax, and repeat.

10. Foot Shuffle (Low Leg, Knee, Hamstrings). Stand back from wall with feet flat on floor. Lean forward, place hands on wall. Shuffle feet back as far as possible, heels on floor. Hold five seconds, relax, and repeat.

11. Hurdle Spread (Back, Hips and Legs). Sit on floor, one leg at right angles to body, inside of knee and thigh on floor. Other leg straight, toes up, back of knee on floor. Move body, chin to knee, hands to toes. Hold five seconds, bounce three times, relax, and repeat.

12. Touch Toes (Back of Legs). Stand erect with legs crossed. Bend forward without bending knees and touch toes. Bounce, relax, change legs, and repeat.

13. Toe Balance (Back of Legs). Place toes on end of step, hold railing for balance. Drop heel as far as possible. Bounce, relax, and repeat.

14. Leg Shake (Legs, Hips, Back). Relax on table on back. Team-mate grasp one ankle and shake with slight pull. Same with other ankle, then with both ankles.

15. Plus the following exercises (Summer Conditioning Program Chapter III): Running, Rope-Skipping, Side Bender, Knee Stretcher, Groin Stretcher, Bicycle Riding, Leg Flexing, Wood Chopper, Quarter Eagles, Trunk Twister, All Fours, Sit-Up and Paw Dirt, Mountain Climber, Leg-Back Stretch, Toe and Heel Dance, Sacrio-illiac Stretch, Leg Stretch, and Groin Stretcher.

### HIP, BACK, ABDOMEN EXERCISES

1. All back and hip exercises in Chapter XI.

2. Exercises number 2, 3, 5, 6, 7, 11, 14 under stretching exercises for leg, groin, hip and back.

3. Hiplifter. On back, feet drawn up to buttocks. Lift hips.

4. Abdominal strengthener. On back, arms across chest. Lift back four inches off floor and hold.

5. Eight Count Leg Lift. On back. On count of one, lift legs two inches off ground and hold; up two more inches on count of two. At count of four, should be at 45 degrees, then open and close the leg eight itmes. Count of five up two more inches; count of eight legs perpendicular, then open and close eight times. By the count go down to 45 degrees and open and close and then on to the floor by the count.

6. Hip Rotator. Inside foot on a book and arm on back of a chair. Outside leg rotates in forward and backward circles.

7. Back Archer. On stomach, back arched, hands behind head. Rock from toes to chin.

8. Bicycling. On back.

9. Pelvic Roller. Standing. Do the hula.

10. Sweat-Your-Shadow. Stand with your back against a wall. Force shoulders, back and hips into wall.

11. Abductor. On mat on right side. Left leg lift from hip as high as possible. Repeat right leg.

12. Spine Bender. On hands and knees. Work spine up and down from hips to neck.

13. Concentric Roller. Weight supported on hands and toes. Roll hips in outward and inward circles.

14. Trunk Twister. Standing with hands behind head, twist trunk to right left and bend forward and backward and sideward.

15. Sit-Ups. Walk on all fours; rowing machine; standing and touch toes.

### NECK EXERCISES

When using weights, use the 10 - 10 - 10 series. Increase weight as tolerated. Raise and lower weight slowly.

1. Neck Flexer. On table on back with body off the table at the shoulder line. Start with head as low as possible and flex neck. Keep shoulders on table throughout exercise. Use weights.

2. Neck Extension. Same position as flexer only on table face down. Shoulders on table throughout exercise.

3. Neck Lateral Flexer. On side, on table. Body off the table at shoulder line. Start with head as low as possible and raise head keeping shoulders on the table throughout exercise. Repeat on other side. Use weights.

4. Dorsal Extension. Face down with body off the table at nipple line. Start with spine flexed (down) and chin protruding. Extend (left) dorsal spine and flex chin toward chest. Do not raise off the table. Use weights.

5. Rotator. On the table on stomach with the body off the table at the shoulder line. Hold head in line with the body and rotate to right and left. Use weights.

## ALL OF ABOVE EXERCISES CAN ALSO BE DONE WITHOUT USING THE WEIGHTS.

6. Towel Resistance. Force head against a towel that has been placed on front, back, and sides of the head. Offer resistance.

7. Hand Resistance. Same as towel resistance only use hands.

8. Rotate and Stretch. Using own hands rotate and stretch neck.

9. Head Glide. Stick chin as far out as possible. Return and repeat.

10. Side-to-Side. Place a book on the floor with forehead on book and weight supported on hands and toes. Rotate head from side to side and forward and backward.

11. Neck Stretcher. With and without rotation, as used in training room.

12. Wrestler's Bridge. Starting position on back, elevate the body and support weight with feet and head. Bridge and turn a half circle. Repeat.

SHOULDER EXERCISES—(May also aid neck)

1. Chair Press. Bend knees so arms are parallel to back of chair. Grasp back of chair and press inward for six seconds.

2. Doorway Press. Stand in doorway, elbows straight. Press outward, six seconds.

3. Table Press. Stand erect. Grasp the corners of a table with arms straight and press inward for six seconds.

4. Ape Drill. Bend trunk forward. Allow shoulder to relax and slowly swing arm in a circular motion—clockwise, counter clockwise, forward, backward, and sideward. May later hold a weight in extended hand.

5. Weights. Use the 10 - 10 - 10 series. Increase weight as tolerated. Raise and lower weight slowly. (Use Weights in Ex. 6-12).

6. Forward Flexer. Raise arm forward, elbow stiff.

7. Arm Raised Sideward. Arm sideward, elbow stiff.

8. Arm Raised Backward. Arm backward, elbow stiff.

9. Shoulder Shrug. Shrug shoulder up, back, and down in a rotary motion. This exercise can also be done without weights —bed drill.

10. Supine Arm Raise. On back on bench with arm to side, raise arm to perpendicular position. Use weights.

11. Prone Arm Raise. On stomach on bench, raise and lower arm slowly holding at 90 degree angle to body. Use weights.

12. Prone Rotation. On stomach on bench, elbow flexed over edge of table, weight in hand, move weight forward, backward, and upward.

13. Wall Weights.

14. Overhead Pulley.

15. Shoulder Wheel.

16. Wall Climb. Injured side to wall. Arm bent, walk arm up wall as high as shoulder will permit by alternately moving the forefinger and second finger. Lower arm in same manner.

17. Towel Slide. Same motion as drying back. One hand above shoulder, one behind opposite hip. Can vary range by adjusting hands on towel; likewise resistance can be changed. Head and neck erect throughout.

18. The Forcer. Palm of hand on back of neck. Lower hand sideward, rotating the arm as it moves down the back until the back of the hand is in contact with the buttocks. The opposite hand then slowly forces hand down buttocks then brings original arm up to middle of the back.

19. Atlas Resister. Force fist into palm of the opposite hand. Offer great resistance with the palm of the hand.

20. Break Chain. Resistive exercise in which you make-believe you are breaking a chain across your chest.

21. Leaning Table. Hands on edge of table, feet well back. Rock from side to side placing weight first on one shoulder then the other.

22. Cross Hang. Hang relaxed from a crossbar. No pull-ups.

23. Push-Ups. (1) Kneeling, (2) regular *with back straight*, and (3) leaning against back of chair or wall.

24. Chair Balance. Support weight between the backs of two chairs.

25. All Fours. Weight on hands and feet, back parallel to floor, head up, walk forward and backward.

26. Back to floor, abdomen flat, weight on hands and feet, walk forward and backward.

27. The Worm. Bend forward placing hands under shoulder (knees straight as possible), descend by walking forward on hands without bending knees until body is parallel and within a few inches of the floor, then walk backward to starting position.

28. Shoulder Roller. Arms to side at shoulder level. Start with small circles (forward and backward, palm up and down) and increase diameter of circle. May also do exercise with arms to front of shoulder, and over head.

29. Shoulder Swing. Straddle position, arms over head, right hand touch outside rear of left heel. Throw opposite arm upward as high as possible. Repeat to other side.

30. Rope-Skipping.   31. Punching Bag.   32. Swimming.

Elbow Exercises

1. Grasp wrist of injured arm. Flex and extend elbow (using force) up to point of pain.

2. Flex and extend elbow with arm in various positions. Thrust hand upward, sideward, forward, etc., full motion, but do not produce pain.

3. Sit on chair. Bend elbow at 90 degrees, rest forearm on thigh, palm up. Rotate forearm to limit of pain, then place palm down on other thigh.

4. Stand two to three feet away from wall. Place hands against wall at shoulder level. Lean forward, permitting body weight to bend the elbows. Then press against wall and push to erect position. As elbow strengthens, move farther from wall. Also do with arm against wall to side of body.

5. On hands and knees lean forward and bend elbows, lowering chest to floor, then push back up.

6. Flex and extend arm in various positions, holding a light weight in the hand. Increase weight as tolerance will permit.

7. Grasp bar (five feet high) and with arms suspended, let the body slack backward so that the weight rests on the heels

(well under the bar). Flex the elbows and pull chin to bar. Part of body weight continues to be supported on the feet. Keep body straight throughout exercise. Use both inward and outward grasp of the hands.

8.   Indian Club Drill. Hold club in and between thumb and first finger. Combine small circles with large circles. The small circles will be above and to the side of the shoulder and will alternate with large shoulder circle.

9.   Trainer holds injured elbow in one hand while fully flexing patient's wrist (palm down) with other hand. From this position, extend the elbow, keeping wrist fully flexed.

10.   With arm first at a 45 degree angle and then at a 90 degree angle, rotate the forearm to right and left with weights.

11.   Pulley Weights. The weight increases with the tolerance of the muscles and joints.

12.   Carry books, etc. in hand of bad elbow.

13.   Bag Punching. As patient nears complete recovery.

14.   Grip piece of sponge rubber (4 by 5 by 1½ inches).

15.   Door Knob Turner. Turn door knob. Bolt tightener.

16.   Horizontal Bar. Support weight on bar and do push-ups.

17.   Chair Bender. Lean on back of chair, and go down by bending elbow.

18.   Pull-Ups. Both with palm out and palm in.

19.   All Fours. Walk in all directions.

20.   Wall Wheel.

21.   Rope-Skip.

22.   Rowing Machine.

23.   Push-Ups.

24.   Darts.


WRIST, HAND AND FINGER EXERCISES

1.   Elbow exercise numbers 3, 4, 5, 12, 13, 18, 19, 21, 22, 24.

2.   Forced Motion. With opposite hand force wrist or fingers, flexion and extension.

3.   Broom Roller. With a broom handle placed on wall at shoulder height, roll handle forward and backward.

4.  Thumb Forcer. With thumb on injured hand, exert pressure on finger tips of same hand.

5.  Spread Fingers. Spread fingers wide and then close into a tight fist.

6.  Sponge Grip. Using a piece of rolled sponge (4 by 5 by ½ inches) grip and release many times throughout the day.

7.  Finger Push-Ups. Push-ups while supporting weight on finger tips. This can be done on floor or against wall.

8.  Wall Walk. Place fingers against wall at shoulder level. Using fingers walk the arm up the wall.

9.  Typing.

*The following may be done with or without weights.*

10.  Pronator Exercise. Prone position. Using a bar with weights on one end, start with arm off the end of a table with weight dropped as low as possible (supination—little finger side down) then pronate until weight is perpendicular to the floor.

11.  Supinator Exercise. Prone position. Just opposite of Pronator Exercise. Start with thumb side down as far as possible, then supinate until weight is perpendicular to the floor.

12.  Ulnar Deviator. Stand with arms at side, thumb forward. Use same bar and weights as for Pronator Exercise. Grasp bar at end with weight dropped below little finger. Lift weight so it will be as close to side back of forearm as possible.

13.  Radial Deviator. Same starting position and bar as Ulnar Deviator. Grasp bar at end with weight dropped below thumb. Lift weight so it will be as close to side front of forearm as possible.

14.  Wrist Flexion. Prone position with hand far enough off table to prevent weights from striking table. Grasp dumb-bell palms up. With wrist dropped slightly, flex the wrist upward to maximum flexion.

15.  Wrist Extension. Same position as Wrist Flexion except palms down. Extend wrist upward until reaching maximum extension.

16.  Wrist Circumductor. Standing. Grasp a dumb-bell and rotate wrist in outward and inward circles.

# CHAPTER XVI

# Miscellaneous Problems
# Related to Athletics

## ADHESIONS

Adhesions are fibrotic structures and are chiefly responsible for most of the permanent disability following operations, fractures, or dislocations. They are formed in and around the muscles, binding fibers and whole muscles alike. If adhesions should occur, there are four approaches to the problem: (1) surgical, (2) passive manipulation, (3) massage, (4) active or passive stretching exercises. Surgery and forceful passive manipulation should be employed only after other measures have been exhausted. Active exercise acts in two ways to combat adhesions: (1) by increasing local blood flow, the tendency toward fibrous tissue formation is reduced; (2) it mechanically stretches and softens the scar tissue.

## AIR AND CAR SICKNESS

Sit in a well-ventilated area with the head held upright against the back of the seat. Eyes may be closed. Sit in the front of the plane or front seat of the car. Prior to departure, take Marezine or Bonamine tablets.

## BOILS

Boils are infections caused by staphylococci bacteria. As an aid in bringing the boil to a head, one may use: Ergophene,

Ichthyammol, Cramergesic Packs, or moist heat. One should not attempt to squeeze out the core. When the boil is ripe, one may spread the boil apart and remove the core with sterile tweezers. Ethyl chloride spray may be used to lessen the pain during the removal of the core. Boils which occur on nose, upper lip or below eye are very serious and should be referred to the physician immediately. More than one boil in the same area is referred to as a carbuncle. Treat all as infections (Chapter VIII).

## BURNS

*First Degree Burns* are superficial and characterized by a reddening of the skin (sunburn, mild scald, etc.). Treat with Nitrotan, Surfadil, Furacin, Salcolan, Sodium Bicarbonate paste, Vaseline, vegetable oils, etc. Prevent the damaged skin from drying out and cracking. (Bear in mind that the degree of the burn may not be evident for 18 to 24 hours.)

*Second Degree Burns* involve deep reddening and blistering—extend into deep layers of skin and do not require skin grafting (severe sunburn, blistering scald, etc.). May require medical care. Treatment: any of the first degree medications; sterile petrolatum; as much fluid by mouth as patient will take. If clothing sticks to burn, do not attempt to remove it. Simply cover with a dry sterile dressing and take to team physician. Opening of blisters is left to the discretion of the physician. Treat for shock and prevention of infection.

*Third Degree Burns* involve the entire skin thickness, with or without charring. Never heals itself, requires surgical care and usually skin grafting. No attempt should be made at treatment, except to remove foreign material and cover with a clean or sterile dressing. Give as much fluid by mouth as patient will take. Remove to hospital in a reclining position with feet elevated. Treat for shock. (Wet dressings of a normal saline solution may be used in an emergency.)

## COLDS

Colds can best be prevented if the athletes will abide by the following rules: (1) Wear a sweat shirt or jacket when not competing. (2) Take a shower after every practice or game, making sure the body and especially the hair is dry before going outdoors. (3) Wear a cap or hat during the winter months. (4) Establish regular bowel movements. (5) Breathe through the nose. (6) Drink plenty of water and fruit juices. (7) Get ten hours of sleep each night. (8) Wear clean equipment.

As an aid in preventing colds, our team physician gives our boys a cold or flu shot before the season opens and we supply Ascorbic Acid Lozenges. To dry up a head cold we use Rhinitis tablets, or if the team physician so recommends, Sudafed. To open up a "stuffy" nose use ½ % Neosynephrine Hydrochloride; Inhalant. To relieve nasal congestion at night, we have used Sprahalant very effectively. Spray in room or on pillow.

### CONSTIPATION

Drink a warm glass of water every day upon arising. Attempt a bowel movement at a regular time each morning. Eat plenty of fruit (prunes every other day during double workouts). If absolutely necessary, take a mild laxative. Massage the colon.

### DIAHRREA

Kaopectate; Pepto-Bismol. The team physician may prescribe Castor Oil or an enema to clean out the bowels, Infantol Pink, Cremosuxidine, or Probanthine shots.

### FAINTING—DIZZINESS

There are many different causes. However, most are due to a stagnation of blood in the legs (standing too long) or an accumulation of blood in the abdominal area (unpleasant disturbance). This causes a circulatory disturbance which in turn prevents enough oxygen from getting to the brain to maintain consciousness. The old method of treatment (head down between the knees) has given way to the more modern treatment of laying the patient flat on his back with the legs elevated. Apply cold applications to head and face. Open windows to get a cool fresh supply of air.

## FROSTBITE

The long recognized method of treatment, rubbing after freezing or rubbing with snow, is no longer the accepted method. The American Red Cross now recommends that the victim should be made warm with extra clothing, and if the injured area is still numb and cold, it should be warmed as rapidly as possible by immersing it momentarily in lukewarm but not hot water. On the other hand, Dr. John T. Phelan of the University of Wisconsin Medical School stated that rapid thawing is the best first treatment because it shortens the time the affected part is exposed to cold and limits tissue injury. He states that rapid warming of the frozen part in a water bath at 109.5 degrees F is the most satisfactory method of treatment. He further states that "increased tissue survival is not obtained when rapid warming is employed at temperatures a few degrees below 109.5 degrees F."

## GANGLION

A swelling of a tendon in which a clear, jelly-like substance (lump) accumulated in the tendon sheath. Usually found on back of wrist or just above instep. Due to an irritation or strain. Treatment: tape a felt pad over the ganglion to help break up the synovial fluid—whirlpool and Cramergesic Packs. Team physician may aspirate and inject with Hydrocortone. Surgery.

## HAY FEVER—ASTHMA

Should be under the care of team physician. When out in bright sun, one should wear dark sunglasses. To aid in sleeping at night spray pillow or room with Sprahalant. To prevent secretions from nose see topic on colds. If an individual has an attack, do not take him into a hot, steamy dressing room; keep him in a well-ventilated room; give oxygen if available; if at night, keep away from cool, damp, night air. Use drugs as prescribed by physician.

## HEADACHE

Many so-called two-a-day headaches are caused by a salt deficiency (see Chapter X—Cramps, Muscular). Other causes are constipation and improper-fitting headgear (see Chapter XIII. How to fit a headgear). Send to physician if headache persists.

HEAT CRAMPS—See Cramps, Muscular, Chapter X.

### HEAT EXHAUSTION

Quite common—less serious.

*Cause*—Hot, humid weather; working in tight heavy clothing; heavy exercise; poor physical condition; overwork; lack of salt and water.

*Recognition*—

Sweating profusely.

May turn into a cold, clammy sweat.

Temperature normal or slightly elevated.

Faint feeling, pale face.

Weak rapid pulse.

Shallow breathing.

Nausea, headache.

Exhaustion, collapse.

Loss of consciousness.

*Treatment*—

Treat for shock.

Elevate legs above head.

Well-ventilated room.

Remove clothing.

Electric fan on patient to cool.

Give saline or quick-acting salt tablets.

Bandage legs from ankles to thigh.

Put in lukewarm shower, clothes and all.

Sponge with ice packs, especially forehead, neck, and wrist.

Ammonia capsule.

Massage extremities lightly.

### HEAT STROKE (SUNSTROKE)

Less common—quite serious.

*Cause*—Hot humid weather; physical exertion; lack of salt and water; direct sun rays; use of alcohol.

*Recognition*—

***No sweating.

***Hot dry skin.

Temperature high—106 to 112.

Chest pains.

Skin flushed, may turn grey (serious).

Strong, rapid pulse.

Labored breathing.

Nausea, headache.

Exhaustion, collapse, convulsions.

Loss of consciousness.

Pupils contract, later dilate.

*Treatment*—

Call or take to doctor (if you take to doctor wrap in wet sheets and keep *cold* on way to hospital).

Cool the individual the best way you can. Put in bathtub full of ice until temperature is at least 100, or wrap in wet sheets and fan, or sit in chair in a cold shower.

Keep in low semi-reclining position (may be too hard on heart to recline completely).

## Impetigo

Impetigo is caused by streptococci or staphylocci bacteria or a combination of both. It is highly contagious and is acquired by direct contact or a lack of skin cleanliness. Recognition is by red spots on the skin (can be anywhere on body, but usually on face, neck, ears, head or hands) which turn into small blisters. These blisters fill with pus then break and form thick, yellowish-red crusts (crusts do not form in infants). Under the crusts are small red ulcers. We have been having success with the following methods of treatment: Soak the area in a Potassium Permanganate or Boric Acid solution for twenty minutes. Cover with Spectrocin or Bacitracin. (Doctor's recommendations: Achromycin, Pan Alba, Phisohex-G-11 Soap or Penicillin, in addition to above.) It may also be treated with ultra-violet lamp or an infra-red lamp directed through a moist towel.

## Insect Bites (bee, wasp, ant, spider, chigger, mosquito)

For any type of bite place an ice pack on it for up to one hour. This will give relief. Other over-all treatment would be to soak in a strong Epsom Salts solution, Caladryl, Ivy Dry, Nitrotan, Calamine Lotion. If pain persists refer to team physician. Also, in chigger bites, cover the area with nail polish or collodion.

## Lime Burns

Wash with soap and water, then thoroughly irrigate with a Boric Acid solution (Cramer's Eye Wash) and apply an ointment as recommended by the team physician. For burns to the eyes, refer to Chapter XI.

## Mononucleosis (Glandular Fever)

Mononucleosis is a virus infection that affects the lymph glands, liver, spleen and blood. The majority of patients are in the age group of 16 to 25. Its cause is unknown. Recognition symptoms are: temperature between 100° and 101°, chills, headache, sore throat, fatigue, swollen lymph glands, especially the cervical glands along side of neck, enlarged spleen, upper eyelids sagging, slow pulse and about five per cent of patients have kidney trouble (jaundice). The illness is over in about six weeks, but it may drag on into years. There is no specific treatment other than sending the patient to a physician immediately.

## PAIN—METHODS OF ALLEVIATING

Ice, Aspirin, Empirin, Ethyl Chloride.

## POISON IVY—OAK

A reddening of the skin with blister formations and intense itching. Wash with laundry soap and allow heavy lather to remain on area for 10-15 minutes before rinsing off. Have all clothing cleaned that has come into contact with the blisters or ivy. To treat, use five per cent solutions of Potassium Permanganate, wet dressing of mild salt solution, Milk of Magnesia, or Epsom Salts. Itching can be relieved by applying: Ivy Dry, Calamine Lotion, or Calodryl. The team physician may recommend Cortisone or Hydrocortisone injections or Antihistamines.

## SCALY ARMPIT, KNEE OR ELBOW

Ultra-violet lamp; Ichthyammol; Sun.

## SHOCK

Refer to Chapter XVI on Fainting.

*Cause*—Injury (self or seeing someone injured); bleeding, exposure to cold; exposure to heat or sun; poison; following operation. May occur immediately or hours later and can be the cause of death.

*Recognition*—Face pale; in severe cases will be dull grey; finger nails and ears blue; eyes glassy, dull, no expression, pupils dilated; cold, clammy skin with fine perspiration on forehead and palm of hands; weak pulse; may have chills; temperature subnormal; takes little interest in what is going on, restless; breathing irregular and shallow; may complain of thirst; nausea and vomiting; may be unconscious; etc.

*Treatment*—Send for physician; place patient on back with feet and legs elevated (head low); keep patient warm; relieve pain or cause of shock; loosen tight clothing; ammonia inhalants; avoid stimulants if shock accompanies hemorrhage, abdominal injury, fractured skull or symptoms of sunstroke. If possible, add sugar or salt (teaspoon to glass of water) to fluids. Orange juice, soft drinks, ginger ale, tea, coffee.

### SORE THROAT

Paint throat with Iotanagen, Nitrotan or Glycerine; spray throat with Merthiolate; Oribiotic chewing gum; gargle with a teaspoon of salt, ½ teaspoon of vinegar to a glass of water; three pints of Stringent to one pint of Nitrotan; ½ teaspoon of salt, ten drops of Iodine, one teaspoon of Boric Acid, ¼ glass of Listerine or Lavoris and fill rest of glass with water; Gar Cap Solution; sip from ½ glass of honey to which has been added ½ glass of lemon juice.

### STALENESS

A mental condition caused by overwork, monotony and boredom. It is usually a personal problem. However, it can affect an entire squad. The athlete who goes stale usually loses interest in his sport; cannot sleep; loses appetite and thus weight; is listless; is tight and irritable and may develop any number of illnesses. He often dreads reporting and dressing for practice. As a matter of fact, he may resent the entire program but will not admit it.

It is the wise coach who will be on the alert for staleness. Following are a few methods of combatting this condition; do not practice too long; do not leave the game on the practice field (see Chapter IV—Practice Routines); change the practice routine from day to day. Add variety, perhaps occasionally substitute volley ball, touch football or a good short swim for your sport; unannounced lay-offs; unannounced special treats (report, no practice and give all a big dish of ice cream, etc.); holiday party for squad, etc.

Staleness is often the cause of the baseball player going into a "slump" or the basketball player who all of a sudden just can't hit. Leaders in industry and business recognize this situation (yearly vacations, long week-ends), but many coaches do not.

SUN BURN—Refer to section on Burns.

SUN STROKE—Refer to section on Heat Exhaustion and Heat Stroke.

## VOMITING

*Cause*—Nervous indigestion; over-exertion; overloaded stomach; not in condition; partly digested food; virus; poison; spoiled food; drinking of milk too close to workout. Any or all of these conditions may cause a condition known as the dry heaves. Presence of blood indicates a hemorrhage. Patient should be taken to a physician.

*Treatment*—If an irritant is suspected, at first encourage vomiting by drinking several glasses of warm salt water or a glass of warm water with ½ teaspoon of sodium bicarbonate.

To stop vomiting, suck a small lump of ice; slowly drink a glass of cold water with lemon in it (no sugar); drink a small glass of water with a teaspoon of spirits of ammonia in it; two to three drops of spirits of peppermint in a glass of water; Pepto-Bismol; Kaopectate; or sip a cola drink.

*Excessive Vomiting*—Have patient sit or lie on right side. Give no fluids other than cracked ice. Apply cold towels to face and hot applications to abdomen. Call a physician.

## WARTS

Many types are thought to be infectious and caused by a virus. They are usually greyish, yellowish or brownish. Some juvenile warts can be removed with salicylic acid ointment or Ultra-sound. They may also be removed surgically, with the electric needle or X-ray by the team physician. See Plantar Warts in Chapter IX.

## WET DRESSINGS

Boric Acid Solution; three parts of Boric Acid to one part Alcohol; Glycerine; Domebro Solution.

# CHAPTER XVII

# Administering a Massage

Massage is the scientific manipulation of the soft tissues of the body. A knowledge of anatomy and physiology is essential if one is going to properly massage an individual. Aimless rubbing may do more harm than good. Unfortunately, the art of massage is becoming a lost one in athletics, primarily because many trainers do not have the time and are thus leaning more and more on automation.

## PHYSIOLOGICAL EFFECTS OF MASSAGE

1. Increases the circulation of the blood and lymph.
2. Breaks up effused matter and hastens its removal (sprain, bruise, fracture).
3. Is a form of passive exercise which prevents muscular atrophy due to an injury and keeps the aged in condition.
4. Invigorates and stimulates the muscles and aids in the removal of the products of fatigue (lactic acid).
5. Aids in stimulation of large bowel (constipation).
6. May be used as a stimulant or sedative of the nerves and as an aid in promoting natural sleep and relief of nervous headache.
7. Adhesions are often prevented. If adhesions are present, massage will aid in their removal.

## FACILITIES

One should work in a clean, well-ventilated room (75 degrees F.) and all massage must be carried out under hygienic conditions. The lubricant used can be most any oil base preparation with an antiseptic content—mineral oil, olive oil, vaseline, etc. or any of the commercial preparations. In massaging the aged (to keep them in condition), many will use talcum powder as a lubricant. The massage table should be of the right height for the operator (so operator can use his shoulders and back while massaging, without undue fatigue) and approximately 20 inches wide. It should be well padded, covered with a sheet, with a pillow available.

## Aids in Massage

1. The complete relaxation of the patient is of utmost importance.

2. Pre-warming (lamps) of the area to be massaged is of great importance. It softens tissues and assures deeper penetration with minimum force.

3. Have a reason to massage. Beware of the "goldbricks."

4. The trainer should:

   a. Be as relaxed as the athlete to prevent fatigue.
   b. Have warm hands, remove rings from fingers.
   c. Strive to develop a soft yet firm touch.
   d. Have a smooth, slow, rhythmic motion.
   e. Swing from the hips as he massages.
   f. Let hands fit the varying contours of the body, with fingers pointed away.
   g. Always support the area to be massaged.
   h. Massage lightly over joints and exposed bones.

5. Do not massage over skin eruptions, infections, breaks in the skin.

6. All procedures should start moderately, build up in force and intensity and end moderately. Do not cause pain.

7. After each part of the body has been massaged (in a full body massage), that portion of the body should be covered with a towel.

8. Always finish massage by rubbing toward the heart. Return venous circulation.

Types of Massage

1. *Effleurage*—is mostly superficial and aids in draining the veins, lymphatics and improves circulation. Using the palmar surface of the hands, apply a firm, even-stroking movement toward the heart. The greater the pressure of the hands, the deeper the effect.

2. *Friction*—aids in breaking up deposits, scar tissue, loosens sore muscles and stimulates muscles and nerves. A circular, rubbing movement with tips of fingers, thumb or palms. Compress the soft tissues on the underlying bone. Use great pressure on adhesions, little pressure on soft tissue.

3. *Petrissage or Kneading*—aids in loosening up muscle and breaks up deposits of foreign matter. This method also increases the blood supply to the deep layers of muscles. (a) Can be deep or superficial. Grasp mass of soft tissue, lift and squeeze simultaneously. Hands work in alternation. (b) Rolling. Grasp whole muscle and roll it on underlying bone, also squeeze and compress. (c) Wringing. Exactly what word implies. Twist and wring the muscle in opposite directions. (d) Shaking. Hand under muscle and shake vigorously (track and for relaxation). (e) Ironing. With palm, compress the soft tissue on underlying bones (chest and back).

4. *Tapotment*—This method is not recommended except in unusual conditions. Tapotment is a stimulating, invigorating, exciting type of massage rarely used in medical massage. A striking movement alternating hands with wrists and fingers relaxed. Springy, elastic blows, not hammerlike. (a) Slapping. Use palmar surface of hands, like slapping one's face. (b) Clapping. This differs from slapping in that one's hands are cupped. (c) Hacking. Separate the fingers, hold loosely and relaxed. Strike with ulnar surface (little finger), giving a vibratory effect. (d) Beating. Close fists and strike with ulnar surface. Make blows elastic.

5. *Vibration*—aids in soothing nerves, increases circulation, and helpful when used on internal, abdominal organs (digestion —constipation). Impart a vibratory effect to the fingers and hands by vigorously shaking the muscles of the arms.

All massage should start with effleurage and should finish with effleurage.

It is rather rare when one is called upon to give a full body massage. This will probably occur only when, because of old age or injury, it is necessary to have a full body massage to keep the muscles in condition. On very rare occasions, one may give a full body massage to aid in the recuperation of a stale athlete. There are many who doubt the benefits of a full body massage in athletics. Drs. Morehouse and Rasch in their recent text, *Scientific Basis of Athletic Training*, made the following statement: "Because of its dubious benefits and the excessive time required to administer a general body massage, this procedure is not ordinarily considered a part of the busy trainer's duties." In the event one is ever called upon to give a full body massage, I feel the formula worked out by Dr. Joseph Dolan is very adequate. His formula is as follows: 15 minutes on lower limbs; 10 minutes on upper limbs; 10 minutes on the back; 5 minutes on the chest and 5 minutes on the abdomen.

In massaging for rehabilitation of an injury, I feel that 12 to 20 minutes is sufficient. In aiding a boy to loosen up before a contest (track), I feel that a one to three minute massage is sufficient, spending a little more time on stretching procedures. A tendency among many is to rub the race out of an individual's legs—in other words, leaving the event in the training room.

A fast-growing practice in athletics is the "buddy system" of pre-game massage. The boys pair off and lightly massage their buddy—after having received the proper instruction from the trainer.

# CHAPTER XVIII

# Artificial Respiration Methods

Artificial respiration should be started when breathing has stopped or when it has become so irregular and shallow as to be ineffectual. Place the patient in the proper position with the head slightly lower than the rest of the body and start getting air into the lungs of the victim immediately. No longer than ten seconds should be spent in preparing the patient. A helper can be assigned to do the following:

1. Call a doctor, First Aid team or fire department.
2. Check to make sure patient has not swallowed his tongue—pull it forward.
3. Remove foreign bodies (chewing gum, false teeth) from patient's mouth.
4. Loosen all tight clothing.
5. Remove wet clothing (if possible) and cover with blankets, papers to keep warm. If possible, apply external heat (hot water bottle, bricks) to patient.

Artificial respiration should be continued without interruption until the victim is breathing normally or until pronounced dead by the physician.

Until recently, the long-established Schafer prone-pressure method had been the method of choice. Research during recent years has been directed toward supplementing the passive expansion of the chest cavity by an actual pull on the intercostal (chest) muscles. This method is known as the Holger-Nielsen method or the back pressure arm lift method (Figure 56).

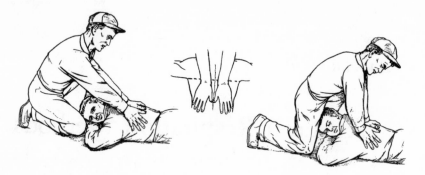

FIGURE 56a. (1) Place the subject face down. Bend his elbows and place his hands one on the other. Turn his face to one side with cheek resting on hand. Operator kneels close to subject—knee near forearm and opposite foot near elbow. Place hands (insert) flat on subject's back with heels just between a line running between armpits. Spread fingers downward and outward with tip of thumbs touching.

(2) Rock forward until arms are approximately vertical and allow your body to exert slow, steady, even downward pressure. Elbows straight.

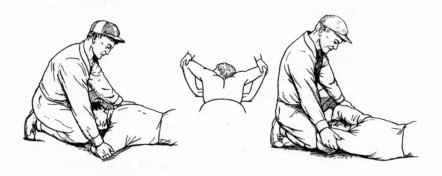

FIGURE 56b. (3) Release pressure and rock slowly backward, placing your hands on subject's arms just above elbows.

(4) Elbows are pulled firmly forward and upward until resistance and tension is felt on subject's shoulders. Then lower the arms to the ground.

*The above cycle should be repeated approximately twelve to fifteen times per minute.

The mouth-to-mouth or mouth-to-airway method of resuscitation is the latest and, at present, considered to be the best method of artificial respiration.

*Mouth-to-Mouth Method* (Figure 57)—Place the victim on his back. If foreign material is visible in his mouth, turn head to side and wipe mouth and throat clean. Insert thumb between victim's teeth, with fingers under jaw. Hold jaw upward and tilt head backward. Close nostrils with other hand. Take a deep breath and place your mouth tightly over victim's mouth and your own thumb. Blow forcefully enough to make his chest move. When chest moves, remove mouth and let him exhale passively. Repeat every three to four seconds.

*Direct Mouth-to-Mouth with Tight Jaw*—Same as above except you may also attempt to force air through nose as well as mouth (especially in small children) and infiltrations should continue every two to three seconds.

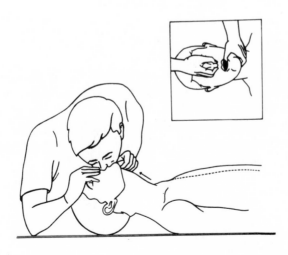

FIGURE 57. Mouth-to-mouth artificial respiration method.

*Mouth-to-Airway*—The Resusitube Airway (Figure 58) has been designed to make mouth-to-mouth breathing easier and more effective. It provides a mouthpiece for the rescuer and a breathing tube which will keep the victim's air passageway open. Technique is same as in mouth-to-mouth method (Figure 59).

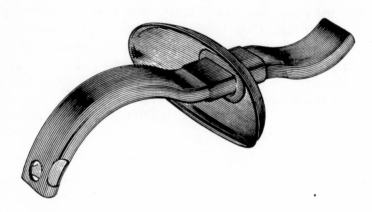

FIGURE 58.  Resusitube Airway.

   In any mouth-to-mouth resuscitation if the air passageway is blocked by improper support of the head or if blowing is too forceful, inflation of the stomach may occur. If the stomach is seen to bulge, stop blowing and press hand between the victim's navel and breastbone. This will cause the patient to "burp."

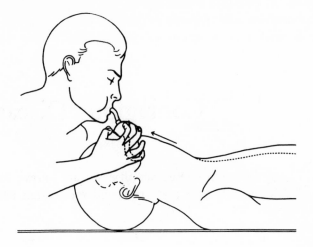

FIGURE 59. Using Resusitube Airway in artificial respiration.

*CHAPTER XIX*

# Contagious Diseases

$M$any common contagious diseases are known to us. I will briefly discuss the four that are found most often among athletes.

MUMPS

*Recognition*—Swelling in front and below lower tip of ear, with headache, chills and possibly a light fever. Bright red pimple on inside of cheek opposite second and third molars. Saliva may be sticky and jaws stiff and painful on movement.

*Method of Infection*—Contact with case or articles freshly soiled by nose or throat discharges from case.

*Isolation*—Until swelling has disappeared.

*Incubation Period*—12 to 21 days.

*Immunization*—Vaccine—good for approximately six months.

*Remarks*—After puberty, the individual contacting mumps should remain in bed because of possible inflammation of the genital organs. Defective hearing may also be an after-effect.

MEASLES

*Recognition*—Begins like a cold in the head with fever, running nose, sneezing, watery inflamed eyes. Rash appears on third or fourth day and consists of irregular groups of dull, red, slightly raised spots, usually seen first on the forehead and face, and spread rapidly over entire body. A positive sign is the Koplik spots which appear early. These are bluish white specks on a red background and are seen on the inside of the cheek opposite the molar teeth.

*Method of Infection*—Contact with case or articles freshly soiled by nose or throat discharges from case.

*Isolation*—Until rash is gone.

*Incubation Period*—Seven to 14 days.

*Immunization*—There is no permanent immunization agent against this disease. The team physician may, however, give shots of Gamma Globulin which has a tendency to modify or possibly prevent an attack.

*Remarks*—A very contagious disease. Resulting complications may be: broncho-pneumonia, tuberculosis, weak eyes, inflammation of the middle ear.

### GERMAN MEASLES

*Recognition*—Illness usually slight. Rash (face, chest) usually first thing noticed. Seldom cold symptoms as with red measles. However, eyes and throat may be slightly inflamed. There may be a slight fever. Glands in back of neck may be swollen.

*Method of Infection*—Contact with case or articles freshly soiled by nose or throat discharges from case.

*Isolation*—Until disappearance of the rash.

*Incubation Period*—Seven to 14 days.

*Immunization*—Gamma Globulin, given by your physician, may lighten or prevent an attack.

*Remarks*—Usually no complications.

### CHICKEN POX

*Recognition*—May have a slight temperature. However, a rash is often the first symptom noted. The rash appears as small pimples which soon become filled with a clear fluid and later become cloudy and tend to dry up rapidly and form scabs. Successive crops of these eruptions may appear up to the seventh or tenth days. The eruption is thickest on parts of the body covered by clothing.

*Method of Infection*—Contact with case or articles freshly soiled by nose, throat or skin discharges from case.

*Isolation*—Until crusts have dried.

*Incubation Period*—Seven to 14 days.

*Immunization*—None.

*Remarks*—When the athlete has apparently recovered, examine his head for overlooked scabs and scales. Seldom any after-effects. *Highly contagious.*

# CHAPTER XX

# Specific Problems
# Related to Basketball,
# Baseball, Track

## BASKETBALL

### PRE-SEASON CONDITIONING

In the modern game, it is essential to get in shape before the season, and then stay in shape throughout the season. Our university basketball season now starts on October 15, and with this date in mind, a player should start to get in shape the first of August. In August, he should work out three to four days a week: jumping rope, distance running, daily exercises (Chapter III—Daily Exercise Program), and weight-lifting three days per week (weight-lifting programs to follow).

In September (first three weeks) work out four to five days a week on the August program with the addition of sprints and basketball drills.

From the fourth week in September to October 15th, one should increase the tempo in everything. Work five to seven days a week with emphasis on rope skipping, sprinting, basketball drills and the above conditioning exercises. By October 15th the boy should be in good enough shape to play a regulation game if it were necessary.

### Pre- and Off-Season Weight-Lifting Program

*Adequate Warm-Up*—Running and rope-skipping are excellent for preparing the body for vigorous physical activity.

*Exercise with Weights Three Times a Week*

*First Week*—Use weight that will permit you to do the exercise 12-15 times without undue strain (three sets, total of 36 to 45 times, resting between each set).

*Second and Following Weeks*—Select weight that will permit ten repetitions maximum. Do three sets, resting between each set, giving a total of thirty lifts. When you can do the exercise 30 times (three sets of ten) increase the amount of weight and continue as above.

1. *Jump Jacket*—a canvas vest in which weight can be varied.
   a. Jump five times as if rebounding (both arms above head).
   b. Jump five times for a jump ball.
   c. Same as above with jump jacket and training spat on feet (weights around ankles which will permit flexion and extension of the ankle).
   d. Ten set-ups with jump jacket on.

2. *Alternate Weight Press*—standing with feet shoulder-width apart, forearms flexed with weights in front of shoulders and palms turned in. Extend right arm upward and return to starting position. Repeat with left arm.

3. *Single Forearm Curl*—Stand with feet shoulder-width apart, arms extended downward holding weights at side of body with palms facing forward. Flex right forearm and raise weight to a position in front of right shoulder. Lower to starting position and repeat with left arm. Keep elbows close to body.

4. *Single Finger and Wrist Curl*—Stand with forearm resting on a platform. Grasp weight, one in each hand (with palm up) and flex and extend wrist.

5. *Double Forearm Curl*—Stand with feet shoulder-width apart, arms extended downward and grasp the bar with palms facing forward. Flex arms and raise weight to a position in front of shoulders. Lower to starting position and repeat.

6. *Sideward Raise*—Stand with arms extended downward and weight in each hand. Simultaneously raise arms sideward and upward until hands are directly above shoulders. Lower and repeat.

7. *Overhead Press*—Stand with feet shoulder-width apart, forearms flexed with weight held at shoulder level, palms facing forward. Press weight above head, keeping elbows straight. Return and repeat.

8. *Heel Raise*—Stand with feet shoulder-width apart, toes on a 2 by 4 and weight held across shoulders, behind neck. Raise up on toes, then drop heels as far down as possible.

9. *Forward Raise*—Stand, arms extended downward, one weight in each hand, palms facing body. Keeping elbows straight raise arms forward until weights are directly above head. Return and repeat.

10. *Walking One-Half Squat*—With weights on shoulders as in heel raise, walk slowly forward and at same time slowly bend knees until thighs are parallel to ground (never below parallel). Continue walking and slowly come up to a standing position.

The feet are very important in all athletics and especially in basketball. It has been my observation that many of the foot problems in basketball are caused by boys' wearing shoes that are too large for them. They should wear two pair of socks (preferably a light pair against the skin and a heavier pair over the light pair), ankle wraps and shoes that fit their feet. In so far as general foot problems of the basketball player are concerned, refer to Chapter IX. Other basketball problems (colds, staleness) may be found in Chapter XVI.

Basketball coaches differ considerably as to the content of the pre-game meal. Some of our outstanding coaches prefer the following: four-ounce steak, tea, toast and honey; fruit cup, roast beef, baked potato, peas, toast and beverage; orange juice, waldorf salad, roast beef, baked potato, toast, honey and hot tea; one sliced fresh orange, toast, honey and hot tea; juice, poached eggs, toast, honey and tea. The above meals are eaten anywhere from two and one half to four and one half hours before game-time.

At the University of Oklahoma, when playing at home, we have our boys eat a regular breakfast and lunch at our training table. If we are traveling, we also try to eat a breakfast and lunch similar to what we would have at home. Our pre-game meal is eaten three and one half hours before game-time and consists of the following:

> Orange juice
> Two halves of a canned peach with natural syrup
> Only two slices of dry toast
> Only two pats of butter
> Honey
> Hot tea

At the beginning of every season we give each squad member a copy of the following advice regarding meals:

### A FEW SUGGESTIONS IN SO FAR AS EATING HABITS ARE CONCERNED ON ALL TRIPS, PLUS THE DAY OF AND DAY PRECEEDING ALL HOME GAMES.

ELIMINATE:

1. All highly seasoned foods (spaghetti, chili, etc.).
2. Highly seasoned condiments (Worcestershire Sauce, mustard, pickles, etc.).
3. Wheat cakes, waffles, French Toast, hot rolls, pie, cake, fried foods, fried potatoes, pork, gravy, nuts, pastries, malts, doughnuts, fat and greasy foods, sausage, etc.
4. Any unusual foods you are not accustomed to eating (seafood, Chinese or Italian foods, etc.).

SALT: Use plenty of salt at all meals and salt tablets before and after every practice.

HONEY: If possible.

TO PREVENT CONSTIPATION: Prunes or prune juice.

IF HUNGRY: Fruit or salads.

* Most athletes have a marked tendency to *overeat*. You will play a much better game if you *undereat* the day before and the day of a game.

* Do not eat yourself out of condition, and out of the league.

* While on the road try to eat the same type and quantity of food as you do the two days prior to a game at home.

## BASEBALL

Probably the most annoying and troublesome injury to a baseball player is arm trouble. However, Peewee Reese and Babe Herman feel that back trouble is the problem that causes most players to have to give up their careers. Others feel it is due to a slowing down of their reflexes or the fact that they are slower in recovering from bruises, strains, and sprains. Regardless of the problem, a ball player has to be in condition if he is going to play to his full capacity, either at the present or in the future. Baseball players, the same as any other, should report the first day of practice in good enough shape to play a game if it were necessary. Our high school and college seasons are very short and as a result the boys have to be ready to play in a short period of time.

### OFF-SEASON ROUTINE

I believe a baseball player would be wise to follow the daily calisthenic program we have outlined in Chapter III with special emphasis on the Wood Chopper and All Fours. Other activities which would prove beneficial are:

1. Once or twice a day hang from a bar (both one and two arms, and *no* pull-ups) to stretch the shoulder girdle. If, after the season, you do nothing, the muscles will contract.

2. Squeeze a piece of rolled sponge rubber (4 by 5 by ½ inches).

3. Run, walk, and play handball, volleyball, golf.

4. Play with a yo-yo, especially pitchers.

5. Push-ups, flat hand and also finger tip.

6. From standing position, touch back of opposite heel, single hand and with both hands (pulley weights).

7. Side-straddle hop, clapping hands over head with elbows straight.

8. Bear Hug. Touch deep on opposite shoulder blades or hug mat or tree.

9. Dynamic Tension. With arms bent, force right fist into left palm (left palm offering resistance). Repeat with left fist.

10. With a heavy ball (not over two lbs.) slowly go through throwing motions.

Continue the above exercises, if you wish, after the season starts, especially the bar hang (#1).

Some coaches do not prefer to have their athletes work with weights. However, I will list a few which have proven to be successful in pre-season work. Keep in mind, weight work is to develop muscle tone and not to develop bulging muscles.

Do each exercise three times a week, with ten repetitions and not more than twenty repetitions with from 15 to not more than 20 lbs. of weight.

1. Single Forearm Curl—(refer to weight program under basketball).

2. Same as exercise Number 1 except starting position is with palm facing the side of the body.

3. Alternate Weight Press (refer to weight program under basketball)—do one day with palms turned in and the next exercise period with palms facing forward.

4. Single Finger and Wrist Curl (refer to weight program under basketball). Alternate: two sessions with palms up and one session with palms down. Pitchers work primarily with palms up and hitters with palms down.

5. Rotator—same as Single Finger and Wrist Curl only start with palm up and rotate until palm is down.

For players other than pitchers, use the thirty-lift maximum method as explained in Chapter XV.

ARM STRETCHING METHODS

Stretching exercises are of vital importance in all athletics, and especially so where the pitcher's arm is concerned. There are many methods of accomplishing this and I will briefly mention a few.

1. Towel Slide—Same motion as drying back. One hand above shoulder, one behind opposite hip. Can vary range and resistance.

2. The Forcer—Palm of hand on back of neck, lower hand down spine, rotate and bring up over shoulder, down under arm-

pit until back of hand is down to buttocks. The opposite hand then slowly forces the hand well below the buttocks.

3. Bar Hang—Grasp overhead bar with one hand and hang, perhaps slightly rotating body. Hang for a minute or so and repeat two or three times. No pull-ups.

4. Shoulder Roller—Arms to side at shoulder level. Start with small circles (forward and backward, palm up and down) and increase diameter of circle. Repeat with arms to front of shoulders and over head.

5. Cardinal Rotator—4 lb. ball in hand. Upper arm to side of body and parallel to ground with elbow bent and forearm perpendicular to ground. Rotate forearm forward and backward.

Don Fauls, Trainer at Florida State University, has had considerable success with the following passive methods of stretching a pitcher's arm. The athlete must be relaxed at all times and the trainer does all the work.

1. Player facing the trainer on left side, head resting on flexed left arm and knees flexed. Place his right arm across your flexed elbow, your right hand on his shoulder blade (scapula) and your left hand on his back (fingers slightly interlacing). Push out with your elbows and in with your hands. Repeat four to five times.

2. Grasp his right wrist in your left hand and your right hand over scapula. Extend or push his arm away from you four or five times.

3. Lift his arm to shoulder level and grasp his wrist with your right hand with your left hand placed on top of his shoulder. From this position, extend his arm over his head four or five times.

4. Raise arm at right angles to body, elbow flexed. Grasp his elbow with your left hand; holding his wrist with your right hand. Rotate his shoulder, both clockwise and counter clockwise ten to 15 times. Your left hand does most of the work as you rotate his shoulder.

5. Player on his back near edge of table, with right arm hanging over the side of the table. Trainer kneels down beside hanging arm and places left arm under his right arm, with your left hand on his chest. Grasp his lower arm, just below the elbow,

with your right hand. Using left arm as a fulcrum, extend his upper arm by pushing with his right hand, being certain that he is feeling the stretch in his interior shoulder muscles, rather than in the elbow.

6. Player on his back, upper arm out to side with elbow flexed. Place your right hand on his wrist and your left hand supporting under his elbow. With your right hand, rotate his elbow.

7. Player on his back. Grasp his wrist with your left hand and your right hand holding his fingers. From this position put his wrist through at full range of motion.

8. From the same position as #7, grasp each of his fingers and stretch them.

At the completion of the above eight passive exercises, with the athlete on his back, grasp his right hand with both your hands and shake his arm four or five times.

Do not vigorously rub the arm before a game or practice. You may apply a little oil, but leave game in the arm.

WARM UP ON THE FIELD

Good legs make good ball players and this requires plenty of running and pepper games.

When a pitcher starts to warm up, I feel that the system a former major leaguer gave me is an excellent one, definitely for pitchers and also for other players. He told me one should start his warm-up by throwing approximately half (30 ft.) the distance from the mound to home plate. At the end of each pitch he should over-exaggerate the follow-through to the extent that he will be able to pick up grass or sand after each throw. Slowly work your way back to the regular pitching distance (60 feet, 6 inches) exaggerating the follow-through until you get to the mound.

All players should have at least two undershirts and shirts so they can change to dry clothing after pre-game practice if they are not playing. This is especially true of pitchers or anyone having arm or shoulder trouble. A pitcher should do his running at the end of practice just before going into the dressing room.

## After the Game—Pitchers

1. Milk the arm—Pitcher on his back with arm raised perpendicular and suspended in an overhead canvas loop. Player may rest in this position or trainer can slowly stroke the arm from the wrist to the shoulder.

2. Finger ladder—Pitcher stands with side to wall and slowly walk fingers up the wall as high as possible.

3. Perhaps massage on off-day.

4. If pitcher has pitched—perhaps a light, quick massage on arm, shoulder and back with alcohol.

## To Prevent a Sore Arm

1. Get legs and body in shape before throwing.

2. Practice your curve ball motion throughout the year by throwing a yo-yo to the ground.

3. Throughout the year, squeeze a piece of sponge rubber (4 by 5 by ½ inches).

4. Wear a wool undershirt at all times with sleeve coming below elbow joint. Have a dry undershirt and jersey to wear if you are not playing.

5. Take salt tablets.

6. Follow arm-stretching methods and off-season practice routines.

7. Many sore arms are due to the fact that an individual tries to really break off a curve ball before his arm is ready. Many throw for a week or so and then all of a sudden cut loose with a curve ball and that is the start of their trouble. Two methods of preventing this that have been highly successful are: (1) On the third or fourth day of throwing, start spinning the ball slightly (goose it up) from ½ way to home plate. (2) Start a slight spin (goose it up) the first day of practice. In each method it is recommended that you make sure you are really ready before you break loose.

8. Dr. Ralph McCarthy, Boston Red Sox Physician, stated that there are probably only three things that help a sore arm: "They are heat plus manipulation, rest, and a sense of determination to pitch."

Sore Back

1. Refer to methods of preventing a sore arm.

2. Very often is caused by throwing against the body (cross fire). Eliminate by opening up the stride, making sure the left leg is out across and to the side when the ball is released. Feet should never be less than in a straight line with the batter. Check with your coach.

Blisters

Other than blisters to the thumb side of the middle finger, baseball injuries have been discussed in previous chapters. To prevent this type of injury, keep the nail filed close to skin, especially on inside, so the nail cannot cut into the skin. This nail should be filed every day before throwing and a nail clipper should never be used. If a blister should develop, open it with a sterile needle and treat as discussed in Chapter VIII. If it is necessary to throw again before the blister is healed, apply collodion for protection. See Baseball Finger and Pitcher's Elbow, Chapter XIV.

## TRACK

Injuries which are common to most track men have been discussed in previous chapters. Therefore, we will not spend any time on these problems in this chapter. Conditioning, on the other hand, is vitally important. I believe this phase of track has been well expressed by our track coach, Bill Carrol. His training program is as follows:

Training is principally an act of faith. The athlete must believe in its efficiency: he *must* believe that through training he will become fitter and stronger. He must be a fanatic for hard work and enthusiastic enough to enjoy it.

There is almost no limit to the achievements of the man who responds *gladly* and *cheerfully* to the rigorous demands of a touch-training schedule, who does not look for a miracle but is patiently content with slow but *well-founded* progress.

The efficiency of a training program is judged by the results it achieves. It is not so much the amount of the improvement, but whether there is any improvement at all.

There should be no hangover effect from the previous day. It is important that you should start each day's session completely refreshed in *body* and *mind*. After each work-out, you should feel pleasantly tired but not exhausted.

The pattern of training is graduated according to severity. First, easy cross-country running for three to four weeks, six to eight miles for distance men, and two to three miles for 440-880 men sprinters, two or three days each week. The results we want in this type of training are (1) development of muscle strength (endurance), and (2) improved breathing (breathing deeply).

After this preliminary period of cross-country running, Fartlek is next logical step. This means *running long distances* (six to eight miles) or as it is stated above for your event, at free, *untimed variation of pace*. It is most effective when the pace is varied frequently from short, sharp sprints to long easy jogs covering 440-880 yards. This should be done for a period of two to three weeks, three to four times weekly.

Our next step is internal running. This involves running accurately measured and timed distances. The principle here is always the same, a fast run followed by a slow run. Each should be accurately timed, and must be kept as closely as possible within predetermined times.

I suggest that distance men begin with internal quarters of 75 seconds, jogging three minutes between. Do at least 15 for 440-880 sprinters, 3x440—75 seconds, rest 15 minutes, 3x150 in 19 seconds. If you get off pace three to five seconds, then you have had enough. If this talls before the suggested number, you will get stronger as you go.

By the time you get on the campus, we will be ready for repetition running. This comprises the running of a given distance in a given time a specified number of times with a complete rest between each run.

*The athlete who has trained hard and consistently during preparation months is able to undertake many more races during the season and his rate of recovery is quicker and more complete.*

# Appendix

## DOCTOR'S RECOMMENDATIONS

ANESTHETICS, LOCAL

Xylocaine—Astra Pharmaceutical Co., Worcester, Mass.
Novocaine—Winthrop Labs, New York

ANTIBIOTICS

Achromycin—American Cyanamid Co., Pearl River, N. Y.

ENZYMES

*Chymotrypsin*

Chymoral—Armour Labs, Kankakee, Ill.
Chymar—Armour Labs, Kankakee, Ill.
Chymar Buccal—Armour Labs, Kankakee, Ill.
Chymar Aqueous—Armour Labs, Kankakee, Ill.
Chymolase—Warren-Teed Products Co., Columbus, Ohio
Orenzyme—National Drug Co., Philadelphia, Pa.

*Hyaluronidase*

Alidase—Searle and Co., Chicago, Ill.
Wyadase—Wyeth Labs, Philadelphia, Pa.
Hyaluronidase Injection—Philadelphia Ampoule Labs, Philadelphia
Hyazyme—Abbott Labs., North Chicago, Ill.

*Streptokinase—Streptodornase*

Varidase (injectable)—Lederle—American Cyanamid Co., Pearl River, N. J.
Varidase Buccal—Lederle—American Cyanamid Co., Pearl River, N. J.

SKELETAL MUSCLE RELAXANTS

Soma—Wallace Labs., New Brunswick, N. J.
Robaxin—Robins Co., Richmond, Va.
Tolseram—Squibb & Sons, New York
Pabrin AC—Wander Co., Lincoln, Neb.

Paraflex—McNeil Labs, Philadelphia, Pa.
Curare (Tubadil)—Endo Labs, Richmond Hills, New York
Trancopal (200 mg)—Winthrop Labs, New York

STEROIDS

Hydrocortone—Upjohn Co., Kalamazoo, Mich.
Hydeltra TBA—Merck, Sharp & Dohme, Philadelphia, Pa.
Acthar-Gel (ACTH)—Armour Labs, Kankakee, Ill.
Cortrophin Zinc (ACTH)—Organon, Orange, N. J.
Hydeltrasol—Upjohn & Co., Kalamazoo, Mich.
Depo-Medrol—Upjohn & Co., Kalamazoo, Mich.
Solu-Cortef—Merck, Sharp & Dohme, Philadelphia, Pa.
Aristocort—Lederle—American Cyanamid Co.,
    Pearl River, N. J.
Kenalog—Squibb & Sons, New York
Cortisone
Hydrocortisone Cream
Hydrocortisone Injections

# MEDICATIONS

Ace Adherent—Becton Dickinson Co., Rutherford, N. J.
Adrenalin Chloride 1:1000—Parke, Davis & Co.,
    Detroit, Mich.
Bacitracin—Eli Lilly Co., Indianapolis, Ind.
Bonnie (Bonamine)—Pfizer Lab., Brooklyn, N. Y.
Butesin-Picrate—Abbott Labs., North Chicago, Ill.
Caladryl—Parke, Davis & Co., Detroit, Mich.
Collyrium-Ephedrine—Wyeth Labs., Philadelphia, Pa.
Cramer Chemical Co., Gardner, Kansas

| | |
|---|---|
| ABA Cold Tablets | Firm Grip Spray |
| Am Caps (ammonia) | Foot & Body Powder |
| Am Spray (ammonia) | Foot Ointment |
| Athletic Liniment | Fungospray |
| Athletic Soap | Gym Freshner Spray |
| Atomic Balm | Hi Score "C" Tablets |
| Atomic Rub Down | Inhalant |
| Butterfly Tablets | Iso-Quin |
| Cramergesic Balm | Nitrotan |
| Dextrotabs with B$_1$ | Nitrotan Spray |
| Eye Wash | Red Hot Ointment |
| Firm Grip | Rosin Bags |

Salt Tablets (impregnated)       Tape Remover
Strawberry Ointment              Tuf Skin
Stringent                        Tuf Skin Spray
Sun Glare Black                  QDA
Sun Screen Lotion                QDA Spray

Cremosuxidine —Merck, Sharp & Dohme, Philadelphia, Pa.
Cuprex—Merck & Co., Rahway, N. J.
Desenex—Wallace & Tiernon Inc., Belleville, N. J.
Domebro Powder—Dome Chemical Co., New York, N. Y.
Empirin—Burroughs Wellcome & Co., Tuckahoe, N. Y.
Ethyl Chloride—Gebauer Chemical Co., Cleveland, Ohio
Ergophene—Upjohn Co., Kalamazoo, Mich.
Fulvacin—Schering Corp., Bloomfield, N. J.
Furacin—Eaton Lab., Norwich, N. Y.
Gar Caps—Wendt Bristol Co., Columbus, Ohio
Gelfoam—Upjohn Co., Kalamazoo, Mich.
Heatex—Taylor Lab., Houston, Tex.
Ichthyammol—Eli Lilly & Co., Indianapolis, Ind.
Iotonagen—Searle & Co., Chicago, Ill.
Ivy Dry—Ivy Corp., Montclair, N. J.
Johnson & Johnson, New Brunswick, N. J.

First Aid Cream                  Resusitube Airway
Nu Gauze Pak                     Scan

Kaopectate—Upjohn Co., Kalamazoo, Mich.
Lavoris—Lavoris Co., Minneapolis, Minn.
Listerine—Lambert Pharmacal Co., Morris Plains, N. J.
Marezine—Burroughs Wellcome Co., Tuckahoe, N. Y.
Merthiolate—Eli Lilly Co., Indianapolis, Ind.
Mexsana Skin Cream—Plough Inc., Memphis, Tenn.
Mycozol—Parke, Davis & Co., Detroit, Mich.
Nupercainal—CIBA, Summit, N. J.
Oribiotic Chewing Gum—White Lab., Kenilworth, N. J.
Pazo—Grove Lab., St. Louis, Mo.
Probanthine—Searle & Co., Chicago, Ill.
Pepto-Bismol—Norwich Pharmaceutical Lab., Norwich, Conn.
Phisohex—6—11 Soap—Winthrop Lab., New York, N. Y.
Pragmatar—Smith, Kline & French Lab., Philadelphia, Pa.
Resi-Film—Squibb & Sons, New York, N. Y.
Rhinitis—Eli Lilly Co., Indianapolis, Ind.
Salacon—Rich & Co., Houston, Tex.
Sopronol Ointment—Wyeth Lab., Philadelphia, Pa.
Sopronol Powder—Wyeth Lab., Philadelphia, Pa.
Spectrocin—Squibb & Sons, New York, N. Y.

Spectrocin Opthalmic Ointment—Squibb & Sons,
   New York, N. Y.
Sudafed—Burroughs Wellcome Co., Tuckahoe, N. Y.
Surfadil—Eli Lilly Co., Indianapolis, Ind.
Tampax—Tampax Inc., Palmer, Mass.
Titralac—Schenley Lab., New York, N. Y.
Unguentine—Norwich Pharmaceutical Co., Norwich, Conn.
Vaseline—Chesebrough Mfg. Co., New York, N. Y.
Vince Tooth Powder—Standard Lab. Inc., Morris Plains, N. J.
Visine—Pfizer Lab., New York, N. Y.
Vitamin A & D Ointment—White Lab., Kenilworth, N. J.
Zinc Oxide—Eli Lilly Co., Indianapolis, Ind.

## EQUIPMENT

Athletic Products Inc., South Bend, Ind.
   Face Mask

Bauer & Black, Chicago, Ill.
   Castex
   Telfa

Bike Web Co., Chicago, Ill.
   Forearm Pads
   Thigh Caps

Camp Co., Jackson, Mich.
   Back Brace

Chattanooga Pharmaceutical Co., Chattanooga, Tenn.
   Hydrocollator

Conco Surgical Products Co., Bridgeport, Conn.
   Alumafoam

Cosby Athletic Outfitters, New York, N. Y.
   Hip Injury Pad
   Low Back Injury Pad
   Thigh Injury Pad

Dennison, C. D. Co., Baltimore, Md.
   Dennison-Wyre Shoulder Vest

De Puy Mfg. Co., Warsaw, Ind.
   Rib Belt

Featherlax Corp., Houston, Texas
   Featherbite Mouth Piece

Gilcrest Co., Kent, Ohio
  Gilcrest Cutters
Logan Inc., Los Angeles, Cal.
  Knee Strengthener
  Shoulder Harness
Marietta Co., Dallas, Texas
  Face Masks
Medco Products Co., Tulsa, Okla.
  Medcollator
M. F. Athletic Co., Riverside, R. I.
  Heel Cup
Mill Mont Co., Long Beach, Cal.
  Mill-Mont Mouth Piece
MacGregor Sports Equipment, Cincinnati, Ohio
  Face Masks
  Face Bars
  Fracture Glove
  Hand Pads
  Hip Injury Pads
  Hip Pads
  Peckham Knee Brace
  Shoulder Pads
  Thigh Injury Pads
  Thigh Pads
O. C. Mfg. Co., Little Falls, N. J.
  Olympic Champion Knee Brace
Rawlings Athletic Equipment, St. Louis, Mo.
  All Purpose Injury Pads
  Clam Knee Brace
  Face Bars
  Face Masks
  Octopus Knee Brace
  Shoulder Pads
  Thigh Pads
Raytheon Mfg. Co., Waltham, Mass.
  Microtherm
Riddell, John T., Co., Chicago, Ill.
  Face Bars
  Headgear
  Headgear Snubber

Scholl Mfg. Co., Chicago, Ill.
Tubegauze
U. S. Rubber Corp., North Kansas City, Mo.
Under Shoulder Pad Protection
Wilson Sporting Goods Co., Chicago, Ill.
Hip Injury Pad
Wolverine Supply Co., Ann Arbor, Mich.
Heel Cup

## PREFIXES

Adero—refers to glands.
Arthro—refers to joints.
Derma—refers to skin.
Dys—disordered, bad.
End—inside.
Hema—refers to blood.
Hydro—refers to water.

Myo—refers to muscle.
Neuro—refers to nerves.
Osted—refers to bone.
Phlebo—refers to veins.
Pyo—refers to pus.
Post—after.
Pre—before.

## SUFFIXES

—algia—pain (neuralgia)
—itis—inflammation (tenosynovitis)
—logy—science (pathology)
—ptosis—falling or sagging (visceroptosis)
—rrhea—discharge (diarrhea)
—osis—abnormal condition (tuberculosis)
—phobia—fear (claustrophobia)
—uria—excreted in urine (albuminuria)
—ectomy—removed (appendectomy)
--stomy—forming artificial opening (colostomy)
—tomy—cutting open of an organ or cavity (tracheotomy)
—lysis—loosening from adhesions (neurolysis).

## MEDICAL AND SURGICAL TERMS

*Abduction*—Movement away from median line.
*Abcess*—Localized collection of pus.
*Adduction*—Movement toward a median line.

*Adhesion*—Abnormal joining of parts together.

*Adipose*—Fat.

*Albuminuria*—Presence of albumin in the urine.

*Analgesia*—Absence of sensitivity to pain.

*Anesthesia*—Absence of sensation (drugs, gas, etc.)

*Antibiotic*—A substance which interferes with the growth of bacteria or viruses, usually derived from other micro-organism (Example—Penicillin).

*Arterial Bleeding*—Bleeding from an artery—spurts.

*Arthrodesis*—Surgical fixation of a joint by fusion of the joint surfaces.

*Arthrolysis*—Operative loosening of adhesions in a joint.

*Asepsis*—Free from infection.

*Atrophy*—Wasting away of a part-cell, tissue or organ.

*Avulsion*—A wrenching away of a part.

*Axilla*—Armpit.

*Bilateral*—Pertaining to both sides of the body.

*Bursa*—Small sac filled with fluid interposed between parts that move upon one another. Prevents wear by friction.

*Butterflies*—upset stomach, caused by nervousness.

*Cartilage*—Gristle-like padding on bones at the joints.

*Cellulitis*—Inflammation of subcutaneous (cellular) tissue. Flat, red, swelling.

*Chronic*—Of long duration, long continued.

*Contra-indicated*—Forbidden by peculiarity of the disease.

*Contusion*—A bruise.

*Counter-irritant*—Product which generates warmth in and beneath the skin by irritating nerve ends, thus causing an increased flow of blood into the area.

*Cyst*—A sac which contains a liquid or a semi-solid.

*Diagnosis*—Recognition of an injury or disease from its symptoms.

*Ecchymosis*—Discoloration of the skin.

*Edema*—A collection of fluid in the tissue.

*Etiology*—Science of causes especially of disease—loosely used to mean "cause".

*Extravasation*—An effusion of fluid into the tissues.

*Fascia*—Fibrous tissue covering muscle and other tissue.

*Fungicide*—Agent that kills fungi and may also destroy bacteria.

*Furunculosis*—A systemic condition favoring boil (furuncle) formation.

*Gastritis*—Inflammation of the stomach.

*Germicide*—An agent that kills bacteria, may also destroy fungi.

*Hematology*—The science of the blood, blood-forming organs and their diseases.

*Hematoma*—A blood tumor.

*Hemorrhage*—Bleeding.

*Hyperemia*—Excessive amount of blood in any given part of the body.

*Insertion*—Point of attachment of a muscle.

*Ligament*—A band of flexible, tough, fibrous tissue connecting the ends of the bones. This is the stabilizing element of the joint or the joint capsule.

*Malignant*—Dangerous to life; invasive of a tumor; tending to invade adjacent tissues and spread to distant parts of the body.

*Meniscus*—Inter-articular fibro-cartilage.

*Muscle Tone*—Normal contractility and promptness with which muscles respond to stimuli.

*Myoma*—Muscle tumor.

*Necrosis*—Death of tissue.

*Neurolysis*—Relieving a nerve from adhesions.

*Neuroma*—Nerve tumor.

*Occulsion*—State of being closed.

*Osteoplathy*—Plastic surgery of the bones.

*Pathogenic*—Disease producing.

*Peritoneum*—Thin membrane covering the abdominal organs and lining the abdominal internal wall.

*Periosteum*—Thin membrane which covers bones and contains nerves and blood vessels.

*Plexus*—A network of interlacing nerves, similar to a cable full of telephone wires (Brachial, Femoral, Sciatic, etc.).

*Prognosis*—A forecast.

*Resection*—Removal of a considerable portion of an organ.

*Sprain*—A twisting of a joint, producing a stretching (strain) or tearing of ligaments.

*Spasm*—An involuntary, sudden contraction of one or more muscles (Example: leg cramps).

*Sterile*—Free from micro-organisms.

*Strain*—Excessive stretching of a part.

*Superficial Injury*—To the surface, generally not below the skin.

*Tendon*—A band of dense, tough, fibrous tissue forming the termination of a muscle and attaching the latter to a bone.

*Therapy*—Science of a medical treatment.

*Trauma*—A direct blow.

*Unhappy Triad*—An injury to the medial ligament, medial cartilage and cruciate ligaments of the knee.

*Unilateral*—One side of the body.

*Venous Bleeding*—Bleeding from a vein (even flow).

*Vesicle*—Small blister or sac containing liquid.

*Viscera*—Large organs contained within the abdominal cavity.

## MEDICAL SIGNS AND SYMBOLS

aa—of each

ac—before meals

ante—before

aq—water

bd—blood pressure

bid—two times daily

c—with

c; w—colored or white

dc; do—discontinue orders

dx—diagnosis

h—hour

hs—at bedtime

iv—intravenous

m. dic—as directed or prescribed

m et n—morning and night

no—number

npo—nothing by mouth

pc—after meals

px—physical exam

qqd—daily

qq. hr.—every hour

qid—four times daily

qsh—every two hours

q 3 h—every three hours

q 4 h—every four hours

rx—treatment or prescription

prn—if necessary

s—without

s or sig—dosage, directions

tid— three times a day.

# Index